Sex Smart

A Sexuality Resource for Teenagers

Sex SMART

501 Reasons to Hold Off on Sex

by Susan Browning Pogány

Fairview Press
Minneapolis

Published by Fairview Press, 2450 Riverside Avenue South, Minneapolis, MN 55454.

Library of Congress Cataloging-in-Publication Data

   Pogány, Susan Browning, 1947–
      Sex smart: 501 reasons to hold off on sex / Susan Browning Pogány.
            p.   cm.
   Includes bibliographical references.
   Summary: Provides straightforward answers to questions teens have about sex, relationships, dating, pregnancy, and sexually transmitted diseases.
      ISBN 1-57749-043-6 (alk. paper)
      1. Sexual ethics for teenagers--Juvenile literature.
2. Teenagers--Sexual behavior--Juvenile literature. 3. Sexual abstinence--Juvenile literature. [1. Sexual ethics.   2. Youth-Sexual behavior.   3. Sexual abstinence.]   I. Title.
HQ35.P55   1998
306.7'0835--dc21   98-19179
                                                              CIP
                                                               AC

First Printing: September 1998

Printed in the United States of America
14 13 12 11   10 9 8 7

Cover design: Laurie Duren

For a free current catalog of Fairview Press titles, call toll-free 1-800-544-8207, or visit our web site at www.Press.Fairview.org

To my brilliant husband, Stefano, who thinks I can do anything; to my wonderful children, Nicholas and Noah, whose births and questions inspired this book; and to my dear parents, William and Peggy Browning, who raised me ever so lovingly, gave me a social conscience, and have always tried to do their small part to change the world.

Contents

Acknowledgments

I am grateful to the many readers who critiqued part or all of the preliminary manuscript: Tina Connolly; Jill Pittman; Patricia and Casey Berner; Elizabeth Jones; Aya and Mina Patterson; Anne Browning Wilson; the Reaumur Donnally family; Susan McDaneld, A.R.N.T., Family Planning/STD Program Charge Nurse, Lawrence-Douglas County (Kansas) Health Department; Margot Breckbill, Chair, Sedgwick County Adolescent Pregnancy Network, lecturer in Human Sexuality at Wichita State University, maternal-child health nurse; Dr. Daryl Lynch, Chief, Section of Adolescent Medicine, Children's Mercy Hospital, Kansas City, Missouri; Dr. Terrance Riordan, M.D., physician of pediatrics and adolescent medicine, Lawrence, Kansas; Dr. Colby Wang, M.D., adult, child, and adolescent neuropsychiatrist, Lawrence, Kansas; Dr. Lisa Berkman, Chair of the Department of Health and Social Behavior, Harvard School of Public Health, Harvard University; Dr. Rita Perll, adolescent psychiatrist, Children's Mercy Hospital; and the author's mother, Peg Browning, who has been active in child support and women's issues in Kansas. I am grateful for their excellent criticisms, suggestions, additions, and deletions.

I also want to acknowledge the important contribution to this book by my sister, Attorney Anne Browning Wilson, who created and wrote the brochure "If We Make a Baby, Do I Have to Pay?" which is reprinted in its entirety in chapter 6. The brochure has been distributed to high schools throughout Kansas.

I warmly thank my husband, Stefano, and my sons, Nicholas and Noah, for their patience and enthusiasm during this project.

Introduction

"My dad gives me this lecture every so often on sex. . . . You know, 'DON'T DO IT!' " says David, seventeen. "But the way I look at it, things are different now than when my parents were young. Now lots of kids my age have sex."

"My friends and I talk about sex, and a couple of girls I know have done it," says fifteen-year-old Talisha. "But I don't know if it's such a great idea at our age. When my mom and I discuss it, I always tell her I'll wait till I'm married, but I'm not sure what I'll do if the right guy comes along. Making love sounds cool."

Sheila, eighteen, states, "I'm gonna do what I'm gonna do. My mom can't watch over me twenty-four hours a day."

"I first had sex when I was fifteen years old. It wasn't for love, just lust. I really regret it and I probably will till my dying day. I really wish that I would have waited." (Teen comment from an Internet forum.)

WHEN IT COMES TO TEEN SEX, TEENAGERS AND THEIR PARENTS OFTEN don't see eye to eye. Parents may skirt the subject of sex with dread and anxiety, while teens wonder what all the alarm is about. When parents do talk to their kids about not having sex, teenagers may act like they're tired of hearing the same old lectures. Yet teens are still nervous about getting in over their heads when it comes to sex and relationships. How can parents and teenagers come closer to understanding each other's point of view? This book is designed to help.

Teenagers see sex as part of their independence, their times, and their rights. When adults urge them to wait, their first thought may be, "What do they know about *my* life, *my* generation, and *my* relationships? Why *shouldn't* kids our age be enjoying sex? We see it on TV, in the movies, in ads—EVERYWHERE! We're nearly grown up. We can handle it. *So what's the big deal?*"

Sex Smart is for teenagers who aren't afraid to learn about the realities of teen sex and to read what other young people have to say about their experiences. The book was created to help teens understand what their parents are trying to tell them when they say, "Sex IS a big deal."

Sex Smart is for parents who don't want to be confused or silent about sex any longer. It can help them advise their kids about a host of sexual issues.

How teens handle their sexuality can be a key

I wrote this book because I remember. I lived through some crazy times as a teenager, and I saw what happened to a lot of great kids. Plus, I've been a newspaper journalist who, over the years, has written about a variety of fixes that people get themselves into when they set aside the rules, morals, and values they've been taught. One of the things I've figured out is that how you handle your sexuality can be a key to how you get through everything else.

Our rush to grow up

Like a lot of my friends when I was a teenager, I sometimes threw myself into situations that I hadn't thought out very well. It was a time of beer bashes, drug use, and sexual promiscuity, a time I survived only because I'm the cautious type. But some of my classmates and friends weren't so lucky. I'm not saying that great numbers of them died in drunken, high-speed crashes, became hopeless druggies, got pregnant, or contracted sexually transmitted diseases. But some did, and these were tragedies. For several, pregnancy and teen motherhood meant the end of what they had worked for and dreamed about. Two close friends had abortions, and one of them still talks of this event with sorrow. I had a good-looking male acquaintance whose face was made hideous for a time by a rash brought on by the sexually transmitted disease syphilis. Two friends died of AIDS.

But for some others, sexual relationships during their teen years left a more subtle mark on their self-esteem, their self-respect, and their lives. These kids figured they'd be able to bounce back unharmed from the breakup of sexual affairs they became involved in. But many of them could not. Those of us who know these people as adults can't help thinking that, if only they had made smarter decisions, their lives would have been much different.

But would they (would *I*) have listened if someone had warned us to slow down in our rush to grow up? What would it have taken to get through to us? Like my friends back then, I was fighting for my freedom, and I wanted to make my own decisions. I knew I was confused about some things, but I was still certain that I could see my life and my choices a lot more clearly than my parents could. My friends and I were ready to take risks, and we threw off all thoughts that anything bad could happen to us.

Why read this book?

So much of our culture—music, television, movies, and magazines—revolves around sex. While much of what young people see, hear, and read seems to blast the message, "Go for it!" teens won't discover the truth about sex from Hollywood or MTV or even from their peers. But they can find it in these pages.

To any teenager who says, "I already know all that stuff," I say, "I dare you. I dare you to keep reading and discover what's out there and what's really ahead for you." This book has the power to make you think, to change your ideas, and to make you look at sex a lot differently than you ever expected.

Sex Smart can help you make intelligent decisions about sex for yourself. In the end, the decision about when you'll begin having sex is yours—yours alone. You will choose the moment. It's your body. It's your life.

Why not just play it by ear?

You may wonder, "Why do I have to make decisions about sex now? Why can't I just wait and see what happens—play it by ear?"

Some young people do just that. They make no decision about how sex fits into their future. Some may "kind of" agree with their parents' rules and their belief that it's a poor idea for teens to have sex. But they feel too uncertain to form their own opinions. When they stumble into an unexpected situation and face an immediate dilemma about "how far to go," they find themselves mixed up and in real trouble. Many let sex "just happen" to them—in the heat of passion, under pressure, on the spur of the moment. And many regret it.

This is sad, because making love is wonderful. It's the ultimate intimacy, something exciting and fun to be enjoyed by partners who share mature understanding, respect, and trust.

If you've always dreamed about how special your first time will be, it's up to you to make sure that it is. Only you can make the decision to save sex until you're old enough to know your own mind, judge other people's characters, and understand relationships. Only you can respect yourself and your future. You, not your friends or your boyfriend or girlfriend, have your best interests at heart. It's important to start thinking NOW about what is right for you.

Finding that someone

If you're like many teenagers, your questions about sex are part of a much bigger question: How do I eventually find someone with whom I can have a lasting relationship in a world so full of loneliness and divorce? It's important to understand that becoming sexually involved as a teenager can actually hurt your chances of finding a long-term partner and having a successful marriage. The pain of failed sexual relationships can damage your self-confidence, making it harder for you to find a strong, mature mate. A dynamic, confident adult man or woman will not be looking for a partner who has messed things up so badly that she or he has sacrificed self-esteem and personal integrity. Teenage girls who have babies and teenage boys who father children are less attractive to future marriage partners. For young men, having to pay child support for eighteen years may scare away potential marriage partners.

Furthermore, sexually transmitted diseases (STDs) can damage your health and your ability to have children. This can make partners think twice about a future with you. It can even cause divorce later—when you and your partner are sick at heart about not being able to have the family you always dreamed about.

All of these issues, plus many others, are more fully explained and described later in this book.

The hardest thing you'll ever do

If you sometimes feel resentful or impatient when your parents give you advice about relationships or sex, keep in mind that they are trying hard to help you. In another ten or fifteen years, you are likely to be a parent yourself. Believe it or not, parenting is probably the hardest thing you'll ever do—harder than getting through high school or college, harder than finding a job and starting a career, harder than finding a mate. As a parent, you will bear the major responsibility for guiding, disciplining, and supervising your children through the milestones of childhood and the mine fields of adolescence. You may find yourself stressing values and morals to kids who would rather keep their fingers in their ears. You will constantly have to remind yourself that, even though your teenagers are making every effort to break away from your control, deep down they still want and need your help.

Right now, your own parents' love and commitment to you run deep; otherwise, they wouldn't struggle so hard to protect you and help you learn to handle your freedom. This book can help you start talking with your parents about your relationships. They can read the book, too, to gain a better understanding of the sexual pressures that a teenager faces today. As alone as you feel sometimes, your parents suffered with these same feelings when they were your age. And chances are they remember it well. They want to help you sort things out, and their wisdom can get you through some tough times. If you choose to leave them out of the picture, you're missing your best source of guidance about relationships and sex.

One teenager offers a bit of advice to parents

A seventeen-year-old from California named Cheris posted this message on an advice forum on the Internet. Many teens share her point of view—even though it's hard for some to admit it:

"As teenagers, we have to make many life-changing decisions that will have a huge impact on our future. Often, we're pressured into making certain choices that aren't exactly what we want for our futures.

"Adults can help us make the decisions by guiding us in the right direction. . . . Having supporting parents helps make the process of becoming an adult much easier. So stick by our sides and let us know you are interested in our futures."

....

chapter 1

Love and Sex

*"Sex is not a three-letter word for love," writes sex educator
Carol Cassell. "Love that is real is a developing emotion,
slow and steady. . . . [It involves] a willingness to invest time
and effort in developing the potential of a relationship."* [1]

*A young man explains, "I thought that sleeping together
would deepen our relationship. But we just didn't know
each other well enough. It turned out we were too different.
I was sorry, and I felt guilty."*

*Twenty-three-year-old Kim recalls, "I was sixteen and a vir-
gin when I started dating Brian. He was great looking, older,
sophisticated. I thought about him every minute. I was completely in love. After a few weeks, we were having sex — in
fact, we did it every time we had a chance to be together.*

*"At first, I was so happy being with him, but then I got
scared and upset. I was afraid he would leave me, and I felt
kind of guilty. Here I was sleeping with this guy, and I was
starting to figure out that he didn't feel about me like I did
about him. I was so sure I loved him, but I realize now that
I didn't really know him. I didn't know then what it means
to really know a guy. The truth is that, after a while, the
biggest thing between us was sex.*

*"One night when he brought me home, he said goodbye in
this kind of heavy, serious way. I could just tell he meant it
was all over. I was so scared, but I couldn't, you know, talk
to him about it. Can you believe it? We'd been intimate sexually all those weeks, and I still couldn't really have an intimate conversation with him about us.*

"For months, I felt awful and depressed. I listened to this suicidal music and stared into space for hours. I was completely confused about who I was and what I had done. . . .

"Then I met Allen. I was so desperate for affection or love or attachment that I started sleeping with him after a couple of weeks. It was exciting for a while, and I told myself I loved him, but I didn't really. I just needed to feel loved. It didn't last long, and I ended up feeling even worse about myself.

"I really wish I hadn't had sex so young. It made me feel bad about myself, and it made me feel like I made stupid decisions. I don't know if I've really gotten over feeling bad about me. I wish I'd waited till I was older."

"JJ" comments on the Internet, "If you can't wait, you don't know what love really is."

FALLING IN LOVE IS FANTASTIC, BUT FALLING IN LOVE CAN BE A MESS. We love being in love. We love that breathless, dizzying, knock-your-socks-off emotional high.

When you fall in love, the ecstasy and the anticipation can consume your every thought. Whether it's a crush, an infatuation, or something deeper, you feel deliciously alive, caught up in a swirl of powerful emotions.

The intensity of these emotions can make it difficult to keep a level head. It's easy to find yourself swept off your feet, sexually excited, and wondering, "Should I or shouldn't I have sex?" At this moment, your emotions are tumbling full tilt, your hormones are racing full throttle, your partner may be urging you on, and there's only that little voice in the back of your mind saying, "Maybe this isn't such a good idea." No wonder so many teenagers take the plunge. Each day, nearly 8,000 teenagers become sexually active.

Some young people think, "Why not? I feel lousy a lot, and sex would make me feel good. I'm lonely a lot, and sex will make me feel like someone cares about me. I'm bored a lot, and sex will be exciting." Others ask, "We're in love, so why not?"

But there's so much more to it than that. Sexually active young people often discover that they're in over their heads, worried, and stressed out. Many teens begin having sex while they're still struggling to answer important questions: How do I know if it's really love? How do I know if it's the right time and the right person? What about the values and morals my parents have always taught me? How do I know if my partner cares for me as much as I care for him or her? What if my partner is more interested in sex than in me? Is sex what I really want out of this relationship, or do I want something more?

Chances are, if you're like many young people, you want something more. What lots of young people are hoping for is a romance full of tenderness and understanding. They're hoping to find a soul mate. The problem with sex is that the focus of the relationship can become SEX, not real emotional intimacy. This makes things difficult. Once you add sex, you could watch the relationship start to fall apart.

And then there are the enormous problems of pregnancy, AIDS, and sexually transmitted diseases.

Before you decide that being madly in love, on top of the world, and made for each other is all you need to start a sexual relationship, here are a few things you should keep in mind.

Does sex lead to happiness?

In books, articles, and interviews with sexually active young people across the country, teens say that sex doesn't make them happy. Certainly it adds excitement, but the final result often seems to be heavy stress, depression, confusion, unhappiness, and, for many, a secret longing to be a virgin after all.

❖

Most teenage girls who have had sex wish they hadn't, according to a survey by *Seventeen* magazine.[2]

❖

In another study, nearly 85 percent of sexually active girls who were surveyed in 1997 believed that they had had sex too young. Half of these girls said they hadn't fully understood all the consequences of sex. They said they realized later that they had not used good judgment.[3]

In a comment on the Internet, an eighteen-year-old girl writes: "A lot of guys don't realize that when a girl steps out after two hours of serious primpage, dressed to kill, and full of lines and moves, it's not because she wants to sleep with someone. Yeah, she's reeking SEX, but what she really wants is to be admired, desired, liked a lot, loved. It sounds corny, but she mainly wants a relationship. What she gets, though, is sex. 'Cause that's what we do these days. Anyway, everybody's doing it, right? Sometimes it just seems weird the way we look for love."

❖

Do you think teens are old enough to have sex responsibly? Are most having sex to express love? If most sexually active young men are both responsible and loving, why do 90 percent of them take off when their girlfriends get pregnant?[4] Sure, sex can be a way to show love, but it doesn't mean much without a real lasting commitment to the one you love.

❖

Michelle, eighteen, says that for some teenagers, sex is "a way to feel needed and wanted even if it's only for a couple of minutes. But when that person leaves, they're going to be alone again, and they're probably going to feel even worse than they did before."[5]

❖

You need to be careful about understanding the difference between sex and your need for affection. You need to remember that the most satisfying parts of a relationship do not involve sex, but are the sharing of activities and time together—sharing your thoughts, being affectionate, talking, laughing, enjoying mutual friends, and feeling that you have a best friend. In fact, focusing on sex could keep you from really getting to know each other. There are lots of ways to be affectionate and close without having sex.

❖

"When Sherita and I are together," says seventeen-year-old Jamal, "we talk a lot. I mean really talk. And we have a lot of fun. I never thought I could feel this close to a girl. A lot of my friends are pushing their girlfriends to have sex all the time, but nothing seems to last. The way I look at it, I don't want to do anything to risk what I have with her."

The sweetest relationship

A young woman wrote to an advice columnist, explaining that over time she had come to realize that adding sex to a relationship can cause pain. She said she lost her virginity as a teenager to a boy who then told her that he already had a girlfriend. In the fifteen years that followed, she had "dozens" of failed sexual relationships. She said she has become wiser and now understands that moving too quickly to sex can result in "pain and loneliness." She describes her current romance as one that involves many hours of talking and laughing and no more than hand-holding. She describes it as "by far the sweetest relationship" she has ever known. [6]

You may be in love many times

The love relationship you're in today is probably not the love of your life. Studies show that most people have seven or eight romances before they marry. You need to ask yourself whether you think making love is truly special or something to do with almost any partner you like a lot.

❖

Love can be pure bliss one day and a disaster the next. One week you think your partner is perfect, and the next week you may be deeply disappointed and aware of their failings. You may go from admiring their every movement to being bugged by just about anything they do. In other words, your attraction can be intense and positive, but your feelings can change quickly.

If you assume that feelings of intense attraction should naturally lead to sex, you may end up mistrusting your judgment.

❖

Many teenagers think that having premarital sex (sex before marriage) isn't a great idea, but they think they might do it anyway if they are passionately "swept away"—that out-of-control feeling when "fireworks explode, waves pound, knees buckle, two hearts beat as one. . . ." [7]

All this sounds exciting, but having sex because you feel swept away is not the same as real love, and it usually does not lead to real love. It can, however, lead to pregnancy, because birth control isn't carefully planned ahead of time.

❖

When teens later realize that their sex partner was not the perfect person they imagined, they may feel awful.

"I always dreamed . . ."

"I always dreamed that I'd meet the perfect guy and that we'd be so much in love and have this wonderful romance," explains seventeen-year-old Sandra. "But I guess I was too anxious to be in love. If a boyfriend would tell me that having sex would deepen our relationship, I went along with it. But I would just end up getting hurt because after we had sex, we would end up having lots of problems and breaking up. This kept on happening to me."

❖

Part of what holds a relationship together is sexual tension. It's true that going ahead and having sex can dissolve your frustration. Yet, at the same time you'll lose the sexual tension that was attracting the two of you to begin with. It's possible that adding sex could hasten a breakup.

❖

Sex educator Carol Cassell explains, "Over and over I hear . . . 'I would have liked the relationship to continue for a while, but once I said yes to sex, it was goodbye. . . .' "[8]

❖

You may think, "So you break up. So what?" But breaking up can be very painful. It usually means that one partner rejects the other. When we are rejected, we realize that someone we love or think is terrific wishes we weren't around anymore. That person no longer wants us or values us. If sex was involved, these feelings of rejection can be extremely intense and painful. They may make us doubt our value. The wound can be deep, and the scar permanent.

As a young person, you need experiences that build you up, not tear you down.

❖

Many teens expect or hope to marry their sex partner. Nationwide, only one out of a hundred high school dating relationships leads to marriage.[9] If you're looking for marriage or a long-term commitment from your lover, why risk your self-esteem and your future on such poor odds?

What is commitment?

What is meant by the word "commitment" when we speak of love? It means a promise of love and caring for another person. It means a promise that you will consistently "be there" for your partner as the two of you live through a future of difficulties and uncertainties. It means your partner can trust your commitment, and you can trust theirs.[10]

❖

When you are a teenager you are just not ready for a commitment like this, even though you may wish for it very much. Teens who think that having sex will result in a serious commitment may be sadly disappointed.

❖

Why aren't teenagers ready for such commitment? A big reason is that as a young person, you are still figuring out who you are. This is your time to experiment with different personalities and behaviors, seek friendships with different kinds of people, try out new ideas, goals, and loyalties. Slowly you will discover what you value, what you believe in, and what you hope to accomplish with your life. These discoveries become part of your self-identity. It's a long process and an important part of maturing.

❖

Until both you and your partner have a more definite self-identity, it isn't possible to form truly intimate, committed relationships. The reason for this is because the "self" that you and your partner are presenting to one another is changing too much from week to week, month to month.

❖

If you hold off on sex, you'll find that each new love relationship can be a healthy step in your search for self-identity. Both you and your partner can grow and learn from the experience. When the relationship breaks up, even though one or both of you may be very sad, both of you will have a clearer idea of what you're looking for in the next partner. You can think of each relationship as a practice or rehearsal for the one that follows as you continue your search over many years for the one relationship that will last. (Also see "Can teen sex affect your later marriage?" on page 118.)

❖

13

By keeping sex out of your teenage relationships, you're doing yourself an all-important favor, protecting your sense of self-confidence and self-worth. Without these it's much harder to form a relationship later on with a strong, confident adult mate. If you're beaten-down and unsure of yourself, will a spirited, dynamic man or woman find you attractive?

Hold on to your dreams

It's important to think now about how you're going to handle sex. It's important to make a plan for holding on to your self-esteem and your dreams. To be in charge of your life later, you have to start learning to take charge now. The decisions and choices you make today set your course for life.

ALL THE WRONG REASONS

Many teens find the sexual experience unhappy because they realize they began having sex for all the wrong reasons. Here are some of them:

- Curiosity—they want to experiment or to get experience
- They want to be cool or popular, or to impress their friends
- As an escape from loneliness
- As an escape from boredom
- As an expression of rebellion or anger toward their parents
- Because they think everyone is doing it
- To keep a girlfriend or boyfriend who is pressuring them
- Boys want to be macho, prove they're men
- Some girls, too, want to show they're tough
- As a means of communication
- Trying to score with as many partners as possible
- They want affection and intimacy
- They're afraid their partner's feelings will be hurt if they say no
- They think their partner will love them more
- They want to prove they're mature
- They want to get it over with

Young people who have sex for these reasons can have an empty, sad experience and may feel ashamed later.

....

chapter 2

How Sex Can Ruin
Your Relationship

*When my son, Noah, was in the fifth grade, he told me that
two of his classmates were "going out." I asked him what
"going out" meant to fifth graders. He thought a few seconds, then replied, "It means they can't talk to each other
anymore. They're too embarrassed. Some kid has to be a
go-between."*

THE STRESS OF A NEW RELATIONSHIP CAN BRING ON SELF-CONSCIOUSNESS—
worries about whether you look good, sound smart, or act cool
enough. When you're a fifth grader like Noah was, self-consciousness kills a relationship dead in its tracks. When you're a teenager,
self-consciousness is at its peak, yet young people try hard to overcome their self-consciousness because they want so much to begin a
real relationship.

However, when sexual intercourse is added to the developing
relationship, things change. Instead of having a chance to learn to
trust and communicate calmly and gradually, partners can find an
unexpected wall of worry and self-consciousness thrown up
between them. The relationship is suddenly pressured, stressful,
and uneasy. Each partner worries about the attractiveness of their
body and whether or not they were any good at sex. Each may
worry intensely that the other will lose interest and break off the
relationship. They worry about the very concrete dangers of pregnancy and disease. They may worry that they are being used for sex
by their partner, that they have made a poor decision, or that they
have done something immoral. As a result of these worries, the
couple may start to distrust each other, misunderstand each other,
pressure each other, and begin arguing. Talking together about real

feelings can become much less comfortable. Romance may take a back seat to all these worries, and a budding friendship may wither. Couples who think sex will add something positive to their relationship may find that the opposite is true.

Not really ready for sex

Kelly, now married and in her mid-twenties, explains, "When I was sixteen, I thought I was ready for sex. I pictured it as being incredibly beautiful, like in the movies, you know, two people so in love, caring about each other, tender, romantic, passionate, all that. I thought if I had sex, it would be like poetry or something. But when Tim and I did it, it didn't make me feel romantic.

"We'd sneak out at night and do it in his car or after school on the family room floor at best friend's house, with his friend outside on the lookout. Not exactly poetic. He started wanting me to do all these things I just wasn't ready for. Can you believe it?—even some stuff at the movies with people all around us. It made me feel slutty. He was having a good time, but I wasn't. He dropped me after a few weeks.

"I think I made a mistake having sex that young. Sex is great now. But at sixteen like I was, you're just asking for a big mess."

Mixed-up emotions

These are some of the emotions that can accompany a teenage sexual relationship: love, guilt, jealousy, possessiveness, embarrassment, confusion, depression, insecurity, fears about sexually transmitted diseases and pregnancy, and expectations of marriage.

❖

Jarod, now eighteen, relates, "I was on the football team, and everyone probably thought I was a sex god or something, but it wasn't true. I was totally inexperienced. I believed in saving it for marriage, but one night Melissa started pushing me. I was afraid she'd think I was a wuss, so I just went along with it, you know, kind of let her do it to me. Being close to her like that got to be the biggest thing in my life. I felt like Melissa was my life. I had this feeling we'd get married when we were older.

"After she broke it off, I couldn't give her up. I kept on calling and driving by her house all the time, even after she started seeing this other guy. I felt so bad I didn't see much point to living."

Sex becomes the focus

When a teenage romance turns sexual, things change. Sex can become the major focus of the relationship. Every time the couple gets a chance to be together, they have sex. There may be less and less meaningful conversation. One or both partners may even plan opportunities for sex instead of dates. A teen on the web puts it bluntly: "With sex, you are consumed by it, and you really can't see and get to know the other person."

❖

Eighteen-year-old Anita explains, "After Juan and I started doing it, we quit going out the way we used to. We'd watch a little TV and have sex. We'd meet and talk for a couple of minutes and have sex. Sure it started out exciting, and at first I loved the closeness and affection, but it was just like lots of things started going wrong.

"I used to think we had something special, and I thought sex would make it better, but it didn't. And I even got bored having sex. He'd be grinding away moaning, 'Oh, baby,' and I'd be thinking about my history project or something. I could hardly wait for it to be over."

Cut off from their old lives

It's common for couples who fall in love to be completely wrapped up in each other—as if the rest of the world didn't exist. But adding sex can intensify their separation from others.

Once sex becomes the focus of their relationship, teens may become even more cut off from their old life and interests. They may find themselves blowing off things they used to care about—friendships, studies, a relationship with their parents. Their friends stop calling because they never have time to spend with them anymore, and they're too tied up to do things with their families.

❖

Sex can get in the way of finding a compatible partner because it can hold a couple together even though they have little else in common.

19

Couples who normally would have broken up and moved on to find more ideal partners may stay together just for the sex—not for real love and not because their personalities mesh. And they may not even realize this is happening. Sex confuses their relationship and their understanding of what each sees in the other.

Dating has a function

Dating is time spent together on a casual, friendly level—without sex. Dating has an important function. It helps you learn about yourself, your needs, what kind of person you get along best with, what you want from a relationship, and what you have to offer a partner. You need this discovery process to build a foundation for adult relationships. When teens move on to sex and sidestep the process of dating, they are risking their chance to really get to know their partner. Just because they're having sex doesn't mean they can communicate maturely. And it doesn't mean they've learned to handle sex in a mature way. Dating a number of partners over many years helps give you that maturity.

❖

Sex is the most intimate form of contact. Why share something so intimate when the two of you haven't yet explored each other's deepest thoughts and feelings over a long period? Sex is not the way to get to know someone better.

❖

How sad to be in a sexual relationship and realize, "We don't really have much to say to each other."

❖

Samantha, seventeen, explains, "I thought I was so ready to find someone to love that I could have this passionate, sexual relationship with. I just had a feeling that it would make me mature, and I thought it would really mean something to feel so loved by another person. But it didn't turn out that way. I ended up sleeping with this guy, Ben, whom I'd had a crush on since freshman year. It happened at a party at my friend Ellie's house when her folks were away. I was sure it was the start of something between us, which is what I wanted, but at school the next week he didn't even want to talk to me. I felt like the worst sleaze. And I was so scared I was pregnant."

20

Being used—a sad lesson

Being sexually exploited—used for another person's sexual plea-sure—is one of life's saddest experiences. For young people, it is a firsthand lesson in the pain of betrayal.

❖

"I figured out that I was just something temporary and exciting for Jerry," says Sarah, eighteen. "But to me, he was the biggest thing in my life, my first love. I gave him my virginity, my heart, every-thing. But he ditched me for some older girl who was better at sex. I know because my friend got it out of him. . . . Guys are mostly players and sh—heads who don't really care about you."

It's sad that someone so young has such an unfair distrust of the entire opposite sex.

❖

Priscilla, seventeen, comments about the pain of failed sexual relationships: "I'm really getting to the point where I don't care anymore. . . . I've gotten kind of numb over the years."[1]

❖

Hector, a high school senior, explains, "As I was growing up, my par-ents, especially my mother, told me that making love was this very special thing. I always figured I'd wait until I was a lot older. But a friend fixed me up with a girl from another school last year, and it happened. This girl and I only went out twice. I hardly knew her, but she came on to me so strong that I kind of stopped using my head. I still can't believe I let myself get pushed into it that way. We were nothing to each other. She just wanted to get laid. I try not to think about it because it still gives me such a bad feeling."

❖

B.J., eighteen, observes, "I've had dates that could have ended in sex if I'd gone along with it. There are girls who want it and expect it. But I really don't want that kind of girl in my life. I'm into girls who take things a lot slower. There are lots of guys like me who see sex as very serious. It's got to mean something. You don't just do it right and left to have a good time. For me, I have to save it for the most special person. I know I'm not going to have sex until later in my life, and I haven't regretted my decision."

Loneliness

Many teenagers feel lonely. A young man confides on an Internet forum, "I'm so lonely. I have nobody. Nobody to talk to when I'm sad, nobody to trust, nobody to love. Today is another lonely day. I'm always asking why are others so happy, in love, and you not?"

❖

Loneliness can be one of the hardest things about this time of your life. Some teens ache for friendship, some for more attention from their parents, some for the affection of a boyfriend or girlfriend. They want to give love and feel loved in return. They want an enduring relationship. The waiting can be frustrating. If you are a lonely teen, when you do finally begin a relationship, don't go overboard in your hopes that "This is it!" Go slowly. Keep sex out of it.

❖

A well-known psychologist comments, "Under the spell of sexual attraction, flattery, loneliness, starlight or whatever, we often manage to convince ourselves that Mr. Wrong is Prince Charming."[2]

❖

The answer to loneliness is not a sexual relationship. A lover cannot create a happier you, except for a short time. Sex could end up causing even more disappointment in your life.

Looking for love is a learning process

It's difficult for teens to accept that the relationship they are presently involved in is not likely to last. We are in love many times over the course of our lives.

One seventeen-year-old named Matt Gibbon illustrates this point in a newspaper column entitled "Teen years 'the best time of life?' Maybe, once they've passed." In it, he writes that a typical teenager's life can be like a soap opera. "So-and-so loves so-and-so. So-and-so breaks up with so-and-so over a silly argument. Mom and Dad deal with the broken-hearted so-and-so for a week or so until another so-and-so comes along."[3]

❖

Teenagers need to remember that when it comes to relationships, they and their partner are still learning.

❖

Sex is not what makes a relationship work. Saying "no" can be the best way to say "I love you."

One-sided love can spell trouble

If the love in a relationship is one-sided, is one partner more likely to be pushed into sex? Yes. The partner who feels most in love and is most desperate to hang on to the relationship is the one most likely to give in to sexual pressure. The partner who doesn't care too much if the relationship fails can dominate.[4]

Partners may have different expectations

Many boys who are in love are deeply considerate and careful not to push sexual activity on their young partners. However, for others the main focus in a relationship is on having sex. They are affectionate toward their girlfriends, but may not feel committed to them and may break off relationships easily and often.

❖

Teenage boys want love and affection, but most don't want to make long-term commitments.

❖

Girls, on the whole, tend to be very emotionally involved in sexual relationships. A girl may see sex as the mark of a long-term commitment to her boyfriend. And she often wants reassurance that he feels the same way. However, if she begins to push her lover over and over to say that he is committed long term to her, the boy may feel too pressured. He may break off their relationship.

Real love

Real love takes time. It involves tender feelings and physical affection, but also much more. It involves respect for each other even though you recognize each other's faults. It involves honesty, trust, unselfish devotion, and admiration that last over a long period. It involves talking seriously about your values and ideals and sharing your goals. It means both partners give of themselves generously. It means supporting each other emotionally and not doing something that will hurt the other person's feelings. It means that each partner puts the other's feelings ahead of their own. And it means one partner doesn't pressure the other to do something they're not ready for. It means both partners want to say "I love you," and, when they do, they mean it. All of these things that make up love take a long time to grow. This doesn't usually happen until couples are in their twenties.

❖

Adding sex to a teenage relationship cannot assure a deeper love, greater faithfulness, or a longer lasting relationship with your partner. Sexual attraction can exist without love.

Pretty soon his friends know all about it

Teenage girls cannot expect their partners to keep quiet about their sexual activity. Sex can cause a lot of hurt when your partner brags to his friends about what the two of you did in private.

❖

If a girl gives in to her boyfriend and has sex, after they break up she may be confused to find his buddies lined up to ask her out, hoping for sex. She soon figures out that the intimate relations she shared with her boyfriend were common knowledge. She feels cheapened and no longer special.

"It took a lot of guts for me to go to school after I found out my boyfriend told his friends about what we did," says one young woman. "I knew the guys were talking about me. It hurt."

Girls gossip about boys, too

Like girls, boys can find themselves the victims of locker-room-type gossip by former girlfriends about their sexual prowess or problems. This can be an extremely embarrassing and hurtful situation for a guy.

Broken-hearted boys suffer intense depression

Sex too young can break a boy's heart. When a young man is deserted by his sexual partner, his suffering may be even more intense than that of a young woman.

❖

"Most of the more seriously broken-hearted teenagers I've seen over the years have been boys. After their fairly long sexual relationships have broken up, these boys become very upset and cannot pull out of it. Some have serious thoughts of suicide," writes psychologist Anthony Wolf.[5]

Although a few members of both sexes attempt suicide after a sexual relationship fails, males are three times as likely to succeed.

❖

Eighteen-year-old Michael talks about the breakup of his sexual relationship: "I love her more than anyone I've ever known. But she won't see me anymore. She told me things weren't working out. Her folks keep telling me to get a grip, but I can't. I try to stop loving her, but I can't. No matter what I do, I still think about her. I can't sleep at night because my mind is filled with things about her. I can't seem to get on with my life."

Teenagers need to understand that adding sex to a relationship can result in unbearably painful emotions when one partner decides to end the affair. The intensity and the intimacy of the sexual experience make you especially vulnerable to emotional hurt.

If you lose faith in yourself

The wounds caused by teenage sexual breakups can make young people worry that they are not worthwhile human beings. If you lose faith in yourself, it can affect your outlook on life.

A young man explains, "After you've had a couple of sexual relationships where you loved someone and they walked out on you, you start to doubt yourself. You start to feel like whatever it is you have to offer just must not be worth much."

❖

A divorced thirty-four-year-old woman recalls, "My ex-husband and I had both been through some painful relationships when we met. I don't think we realized it at the time, but what we had most in common was that we felt so lost. Neither one of us had much self-esteem. We kind of clung to each other in desperation, I guess.

"After we got married, we started to realize that we each had completely different ideas about how to handle our lives and our marriage, and we started to kind of go our own ways. Three years and two kids later, we were divorced. It's been rough. Sometimes I think that if I hadn't been so anxious to get into sexual relationships when I was younger, I'd have been a different person, a stronger person. And I might have made a different choice when it came to choosing a husband. My ex probably feels the same way."

Your sense of self-worth

In a book called *Men Like Women Who Like Themselves*, Steven Carter and Julia Sokol state that "The Smartest Woman is a woman who has a clear, indisputable sense of her worth. . . ."[6]

Unfortunately, your sense of self-worth takes a real tumble when you are rejected by sex partners. It's hard to get over feeling bad about yourself. This is just as true for boys and young men.

When you break up

The breakup of a sexual relationship can be so overwhelming that a teenager can concentrate on little else. School work begins to slide, and that only makes things worse.

❖

Teens may have lost the support of friends at a time when they need it the most. While they were so wrapped up in their sexual partner, their best friends may have felt abandoned—and found new friends.

❖

When sexual relationships break up, teens often feel rejected and hurt. Desperate for affection, they may find themselves falling into bed with the next person who comes along and treats them well. It can become a vicious cycle of affection-sex-rejection-hurt.

Why would he dump her after sex?

Rina, eighteen, says, "Every time Angelo and I went out, he was all over me to make love with him. He kept saying we loved each other and it would be a sign of our love, and he wore down my resistance. After we made love a few times, he told me he didn't think our relationship was going anywhere and he dumped me. Just like that. Can you believe it? I felt like dirt."

Why do counselors hear this story so often? A girl dates a guy for several weeks and really likes him. He tells her he has strong feelings for her, she has sex with him, and he soon tells her he wants to break off the relationship.

❖

Often it's the boy who talked the girl into having sex, so why does he drop her when she's taken such a big step and has done what he asked? In the following excerpts, some boys explain why.

- "I know I pushed Crystal pretty hard," recalls Joe. "But when she gave in, I had this feeling that if she'd do it with me, she'd probably do it with lots of guys. I just didn't feel the same about her after that."

- Jim explained, "I can't help it if it makes me sound bad, but I just got bored with Dana."

- "Julie keeps pushing me to tell her I love her and that I won't go out with anyone but her," says Nick. "She keeps talking about getting married. Geez, I'm seventeen and she thinks I'm gonna tell her we'll be together forever? No way."

- "As soon as we did it," says Kent, "everything started going wrong. I didn't know it was going to be such a big thing to her. She kept saying she was worried that she shouldn't have done it, that her virginity was this big deal, and was I sure I loved her. I didn't mean to hurt her feelings. I liked her okay, but I couldn't handle how guilty she made me feel. I finally got mad at her and we had this big fight about it and I said I thought we should call it off. She kind of freaked. The whole thing made me feel awful. I was sorry for her, but I was glad it was over. I just felt this weight off me."

Does it mean your partner is a jerk?

The truth is that most boys who break up a sexual relationship in a cruel way are not jerks. Nor are the girls who hurt boys. They are just in over their heads. Most hurt one another without understanding the damage they are doing. Young people who start having sex and think they can handle it with maturity may be asking too much of themselves.

Sex can be a trap

The following is a letter to Ann Landers:

Dear Ann:

I've gotten myself into a mess. I'm a sixteen-year-old girl who is having sex with my boyfriend, who is eighteen. I'll call him Ed. I'm what you'd call a nice girl, I think. I don't smoke or do drugs or any of that stuff. My grades are good.

After Ed and I had been dating for a few months, it just seemed natural to have sex with him. He didn't pressure me. I wanted it as much as he did. We're using birth control pills and condoms, so I'm not worried about getting pregnant. What I'm worried about is how I feel now about Ed and me. I don't want to keep on doing this. I told Ed I want to stop, but he doesn't. I don't enjoy going out with him anymore because I know every date will mean more sex. My parents know what's going on, and my dad can hardly look at me. The other day, he said he wanted to have Ed arrested for statutory rape. Some days, I wish he would. It looks as if it's the only way I can get out of this situation.

I thought I was in love with Ed, but now I know it was more physical than anything else. I had heard people say it's dumb to have sex at my age, but I wouldn't listen. I'd do anything to undo what I've done. Please, Ann, keep telling people what a big mistake it is to have sex too soon. If only one girl like me listens, it will be worth the pain I went through to write this letter.

—Missy [7]

Missy realized that she confused sexual attraction with love. Her sexual relationship with Ed has damaged her feelings for him completely, and she feels hopelessly trapped. If she didn't feel pressured to begin having sex, she certainly feels pressured now. She worries about what her parents think of her. She understands how badly Ed will be hurt if she breaks off their relationship, and she can't face doing it. Missy and Ed are in over their heads. Missy desperately wishes she'd never started having sex. She wishes she were happy again.

Strengthen your relationship — keep sex out of it

Most teenagers are confused and worried about sex. Chances are good they'll admire a partner with self-respect and sexual integrity. If your partner is worthy of your trust and affection, and if they really care about you, they'll respect your decision to hold off on sex. They may actually be relieved.

❖

If your partner ends the relationship over sex, they were clearly NOT someone you could have counted on anyway.

❖

If you keep sex out of your relationship, you and your partner may be more likely to develop a lasting friendship, respect, trust, and understanding. Even if the two of you break up and seek new partners, you won't see the relationship as a black mark that stains your self-image and your pride.

"SEX!"

Sure, it's hard to stop thinking about sex and imagining what it's like. After all, your hormones are screaming "SEX!" It's normal to have thoughts and fantasies about sex, but you also need to listen to that voice inside you that says, "Yeah, I'm curious, but sex will still be there when I'm older. Why make my life any more complicated than it is right now? I've got enough to worry about without getting in over my head with sex."

29

····················

Are Males and Females on the Same Sexual "Wavelength"?

"I used to try to get all my girlfriends into bed," recalls nineteen-year-old Richard. "I didn't think much of it. I was having fun. But I saw things kind of differently after my little sister fell for this dweeb and started sleeping with him. When he dumped her, it really screwed up her life. She was only sixteen, just a kid. It made me see that girls don't look at sex the same as guys."

On the Internet, a young man named Scott gives his opinion and some advice to young women: "Women are affected more by their emotions than guys. . . . Keep your guard up. If you can keep your senses and play it smart, you can enjoy the differences in the sexes and not just get hurt by them. Guys aren't going to think like you do. Don't expect them to." [1]

WHEN IT COMES TO SEXUAL APPETITES AND WHAT WE LOOK FOR IN A sexual relationship, there are some big differences between males and females. It is important to understand these differences. The idea is not to put blame on one sex or the other for their behavior, but to understand each other's behavior within a relationship. The more you understand, the less likely you'll be confused or hurt.

The hormones kick in

Testosterone is the sex hormone for both males and females. It is also thought to be the hormone of aggression and dominance.

After puberty, boys have twenty times as much testosterone in their bodies as girls. It is believed that all this testosterone makes boys more sexually aware and sexually active than girls.[2]

❖

Teenage boys are at the height of their sex drive. On the other hand, girls don't reach their sexual peak until they're around thirty. Therefore, most teenage girls don't feel the same strong need for sex as boys.

Are we "created equal" when it comes to sex?

Men and women are not created equal sexually. Our differences go beyond genital differences. The brains of men and women process information differently, leading to different ways of understanding and behaving.[3]

❖

According to sociologist David Popenoe, "Males are more sexually driven and promiscuous while females are more relationship-oriented, thus setting up a continuous tension between the sexes."[4]

❖

"Girls look for security, and boys seek adventure. Boys are after variety, and girls want intimacy," writes Barbara Dafoe Whitehead, social historian.[5]

❖

Lots of girls are raised to believe that sex is tied to love and romance. Lots of boys, on the other hand, are conditioned to separate love from sex and physical pleasure. Some boys are pushed by their friends to believe that "scoring" is what counts.

❖

From an early age, many girls fantasize about the wonders of being in love. On the other hand, many boys tease each other mercilessly about being in love, as if it's something only a sissy would feel. Yet some boys urge others to get all the sex they can.

❖

In their relationships, many young men and women look for warmth, sensitivity, communion, company, and emotional contact. Yet, many girls may be satisfied with touching, embracing, and kissing a boy, while lots of boys would like the physical affection to lead to sexual intercourse.[6]

❖

Unless young people understand these big differences, they're likely to hurt one another.

❖

According to a survey by *Seventeen* magazine and the Ms. Foundation, many girls behave aggressively because they want so much to be asked out. "But when it comes to sex, it is the boys who are pushing for it." Nearly three-fourths of the girls questioned said they only had sex because their boyfriends pressured them.[7]

Most girls want affection more than sex

After interviewing hundreds of girls, Lesley Jane Nonkin Seymour, editor-in-chief of *YM* magazine, says that nearly all the girls she talked with preferred "emotionally fulfilling affection" over sex. In her book, *I Wish My Parents Understood*, she quotes a fifteen-year-old girl: "Sometimes you can picture yourself being with a guy, but it's never to the physical extent. Girls just aren't like guys; they don't need to get laid."[8]

❖

A seventeen-year-old girl observes, "You're first attracted to a guy by what he looks like. I guess that might be subconsciously related to sex, but we don't really think of it that way. We think, oh, he's so cute, he's so adorable—not about whether we can make out or get down to it with him."[9]

Lots of boys—but not all—feel the same way about girls

Dr. Ruth Westheimer quotes two boys in her book *First Love*.[10]

One says, "When I make out with someone, it's physical. I don't want to talk about love. I might pretend it's love because they want me to, but really I want to fool around. And I think about going the whole way all the time."

Another admits, "When I look at girls or think about them, I think about their bodies and sex. I know what they mean about love, but I have to admit I don't really feel that."

Different reactions to body changes

Boys and girls experience physical changes during their early teen years. But these changes affect the two sexes psychologically in different ways. As their body weight increases, boys tend to feel more powerful and dominant. But as body weight increases in girls, they may begin to feel anxious, gross, or disgusted with themselves. Unfortunately, our culture is obsessed with thinness. Instead of feeling more powerful as they develop, girls may feel less sure of themselves and more insecure in relationships with boys.[11] As a result, it can be harder for them to say no when boys are aggressive about wanting to have sex.

What does "I love you" mean?

To get sex, a boy may untruthfully tell a girl what she wants so much to hear—that he loves her. He may tell her he will love her even more if she has sex with him. Girls are ready to believe this. Boys need to realize how devastated a girl will be later when she realizes that her trust was misplaced.

❖

Girls should remember that some boys use the word "love" because they want to become sexually involved. And some boys say "love" when they really mean "like."

❖

Sex educator and author Cynthia Akagi explains that boys often say "I love you" when they mean:
- "I like you a lot."
- "I love you right now when we're together but not forever."
- "I love you so I can make out or have sex with you."

She says some boys are not necessarily trying to trick a girl when they say "I love you." They think it's what they're supposed to say.[12]

❖

Akagi describes a study of high school boys. Ninety percent of these boys said they would tell a girl just about anything to get her to make out or have sex with them. Some of the boys said they "didn't like themselves" for this dishonesty.[13]

❖

Boys need to remember that using love to bargain for sex is not only dishonorable and breaks girls' hearts, but it also damages a boy's own positive sense of the kind of guy he is. In other words, this behavior robs him of his own self-respect. Only by respecting others can you feel respect for yourself.

❖

"When I was young, I ruined a lot of relationships by pushing so hard for sex," recalls a married man. "I'm kind of ashamed when I look back on it. Sure, I took girls out for dinner or to a movie . . . but my main goal was to get them into bed. I pushed pretty hard. Lots of nice girls didn't want to go out with me after a few dates. When I look back on it, I'm embarrassed about what they must have thought of me."

What about girls who push for sex?

"There's this girl who's starting to talk to me all the time at school," says Ben, fifteen. I've heard some rumors about her and her last boyfriend having sex. The other day in math she wrote her name and phone number on my hand. I like her but I'm scared of the way she's acting and kind of expecting me to talk sexy to her."

❖

Although most girls prefer affection to sex, some guys these days are surprised to find themselves getting pressured for sex by girls. This can be the result of a girl's high sex drive, curiosity, pressure from her peers, her need to feel loved, her confusing sex with love, or her notion that sex is how you attract and hold on to a boyfriend. A few girls measure their self-esteem by the number of boys they sleep with. Some want to tie themselves to a guy by any means possible. Guys, like girls, need to be careful not to allow themselves to be pushed into sex.

Different ways of looking at sex and marriage

It is common for young women in high school and college who are in a sexual relationship to have expectations of marriage. But many young men do not see a sexual affair as necessarily leading to marriage. Most don't consider getting married until they've completed high school and college and have started a career.

Leaving love behind

For guys with big dreams for the future, getting well established in a career is the number one objective. If they must move far away to go to school or get a job, they are ready to give up love relationships to further their career.

"It's clear to me that I don't really have a choice," says a young man who is leaving behind a serious relationship to attend school in a distant state. "My goals are what count right now. Leaving my girlfriend is a small sacrifice for the future. After I get this behind me, then I can focus on a relationship and love."

Many young women would not leave love behind like this, although this is slowly beginning to change. They would be more apt to do the opposite—sacrifice a smart career move for love. Young women might want to remember this difference between the sexes when they're considering becoming sexually involved and expecting that a long-term or permanent commitment will follow.

❖

"It's crazy to think that our relationship is going to continue into college," says Louis, a high school senior. Although he has been involved in a serious relationship with his girlfriend for two years, he explains, "I feel like the future is just opening up."

What is a romantic act?

Researchers at one university asked college students what they considered to be a "romantic act." Both men and women mentioned things like taking walks together, giving or receiving flowers, or a candlelight dinner. However, women often mentioned hearing "I love you" as romantic, while men hardly named this. And men mentioned having sex as an act of romance, while women did not.[14] This points to a very big difference between young men and women.

How it is for guys

Psychologist Dr. Archibald Hart says that nature programs men with an almost irresistible urge for sex. Men love sex, are designed for sex, and feel such strong impulses and desires for sex that they sometimes think they're "going crazy." Yet, Hart says, these male feelings are usually quite normal. [15]

A fifteen-year-old girl named Jerry would agree. She laughs, "Guys are mostly interested in sex. . . . I mean, if a guy sees a girl walking down the street he's not going to think, 'Oh, what a mind!' . . . He'll look at her body and think, 'Oh, wow, I'd like to—!' " [16]

❖

One of the reasons boys think this way is that lots of girls these days act sexy and dress in sexy or revealing clothing that is intended to make them desirable to boys. While what these girls mostly want is to have a boyfriend, many boys get the message that girls are sexually available.

Scoring

Some guys feel an urge for sexual conquest and variety that leads to what is called "scoring," trying to have sex with as many girls as possible. Because some boys are so eager to score, they come to view girls as "sex objects." In other words, they think girls are what you use to get sex.

Ben Franklin talked about it

The desire for variety is nothing new. Even the esteemed Benjamin Franklin said in his *Almanack*, "After three days men grow weary of a wench, a guest, and weather rainy." [17]

But boys need love and affection, too

But while they're acting like studs, what's really going on in most boys' heads? Of his own experience growing up, Dr. Robert Pasick, a psychotherapist and author, writes that most boys he knew tried to act confident and savvy about sex, but, in reality, most were bewildered and felt like "lost little boys." [18]

❖

Like girls, most teenage boys want love, affection, intimacy, and tenderness. Yet many boys can enjoy sex without feeling that they need a lengthy commitment. However, because so many girls believe that sex must be the mark of a deep, long-term commitment that might lead to marriage, there are bound to be disappointed girls with broken hearts and shattered self-esteem. Boys may end up feeling guilty. Some may feel angry about feeling guilty.

Will things ever change?

These differences illustrate why teenage sexual relationships often end badly and why the "next" sexual relationship may suffer from the same problems as the last one. These are differences we can't change. If young couples keep sex out of it, their misunderstandings over commitment are not so devastating. And in many cases, their relationships may last longer because there is more real understanding and less stress, distrust, and argument.

❖

Neil, seventeen, says he's decided to keep sex out of his dating relationships. He observes, "I'm not in a hurry. I'm good friends with lots of girls and that's the way I like it. The idea of having sex is exciting I guess, but when I look at some of the messed up, weirded out guys I know who had sex with their girlfriends and broke up, I figure who needs that kind of excitement? I think I've had more fun in high school than lots of guys I know."

❖

By postponing sex, teens avoid self-destructive behaviors and give each other a chance to grow up and face relationships with maturity.

❖

When a man is in his twenties, he thinks more seriously about settling down, and he gains a greater sensitivity to a woman's feelings and needs. He gains a more mature sense of duty and loyalty. He makes "an effort to construct a life of purpose, decency, and productivity."[19] At this age, a young woman and young man are better able to judge and understand each other's deeper character. This coincides with the age at which most people choose a lifetime partner.

chapter 4

....

"It Wasn't at All
What I Expected"

A nineteen-year-old comments, "Everyone's going around wondering why they aren't having the greatest sexual experiences in the world and nobody's saying anything about it." [1]

One seventeen-year-old girl remembers, "The first time I had intercourse I was lying there thinking, You mean this was IT? Am I supposed to be thrilled by this? It wasn't that it hurt me or anything, because it didn't. It just didn't feel like anything to me. I figured there must be something wrong with me, so I didn't say a word to him." [2]

Asked to describe the feelings that led to her first sexual encounter, a nineteen-year-old recalled, "My boyfriend and I were kissing and touching, you know, and I was so caught up in it . . . like nothing existed except him and me. It was like total excitement and total fear. The feeling was so intense.

"But then we did it, we made love, and then there was . . . just nothing. All that excitement, then only this short physical act that was just kind of nothing. I didn't know what to think."

An advice columnist for a teen magazine says, "We often get letters from girls who had sex, had a lousy experience, and wish they hadn't done it."

TEENAGERS ARE HAVING SEX AT YOUNGER AND YOUNGER AGES COMPARED with previous generations.[3] But many discover that sex has been vastly overrated. Young people of both sexes are finding sex to be disappointing, dissatisfying, and even depressing. After experiencing something that was supposed to be incredibly special and fulfilling, many think, "It wasn't at all what I expected."

Popular music, TV, movies, and advertising make it sound like sex is the most terrific and glorious thing two people can share. You may think that if you have sex, you'll move into some sophisticated new phase of life. Sex can't accomplish this. Even in a great marriage, sex is only a small part of a couple's life together.

For married couples, sex is an exciting and pleasurable physical activity based on a history of understanding, trust, love, and respect. Married couples have had time to work at understanding each other's sexual needs. Sex is meaningful because the relationship is meaningful—the relationship has withstood the test of time.

Without this commitment and respect, sex is a shallow, unfulfilling, physical act. And without excellent communication and a clear understanding of each other's sexual needs, sex isn't even likely to feel good—especially for girls. Intercourse among young teens has been described as "nasty, brutish, and short."[4] No wonder so many teens are disappointed.

By the time they're married, they may not care too much for sex anymore. Their experiences may have been so negative and depressing that sex has lost its charm and excitement. By giving in to sex too young, teens may cheat themselves out of the sense of joy and specialness of sex with a lifetime partner.

I've been waiting all this time for THAT?

Sexually active teens don't realize that truly satisfying sex will probably not occur until they're older. Here they have taken the plunge, crossed the final frontier, and it was a dud. Sex was a mechanical act followed by a feeling of loneliness.

❖

During sexual intercourse, most boys are not concerned with what the girl is going through or the quality of her experience. Some girls experience fear, pain, trauma—not pleasure or orgasm (the height of sensation of sexual pleasure).

❖

Looking back, a man named Eliot recalls, "When I was first starting off to have sex, it was real straightforward: get a hard-on, stick it in, come, and that's that. It was a real selfish thing. . . . It's like proving something to yourself and to the world: I'm a man, I have sex, I come. But actually, even though I was physically getting off, I wasn't really enjoying sex the way I had fantasized it would be. I had a nagging suspicion that I wasn't really making love, you know. I didn't know anything about how to give someone else pleasure, and what was worse, I didn't even know that there was anything to know."[5]

He thinks it's her problem

The average boy has no idea about what it takes for a female to have a satisfying sexual experience. He just figures that if he reaches orgasm and she doesn't, it's her problem. Most young girls do not experience orgasm, but they are too shy to tell their partners that they are getting nothing out of the experience. To please boyfriends, many girls fake having an orgasm. No wonder so many are sad and sorry that they gave up their virginity so easily. If they had waited until they were in a trusting, long-term relationship like marriage, they would have found themselves better able to talk over their sexual needs with their partner to achieve mutual pleasure. Discussing sexual needs is just too excruciatingly embarrassing for most teens to deal with.

❖

Lots of young people pretend they enjoy sex when in fact they really don't. Girls, confused and disappointed, lie to their partner and friends about their level of enjoyment.

❖

According to columnist Ann Landers, "Often girls write to tell me of their deep disappointment. They thought it was going to be the most glorious thing that ever happened, but instead it made them feel cheap, dirty and disgusted with the boy as well as with themselves."[6]

❖

When a boy senses his partner's disappointment, he may secretly feel that he is a failure or that he is not a real man.

Will it be romantic?

Deep in the hearts and minds of many teenagers is a vision of how their first sexual experience will be. They picture a loving partner, a beautiful place, an aura of romance. Here is the reality of where most teenage sexual encounters occur:

- In a car, sometimes with another couple present
- On the floor
- At night in a public place, which can be dangerous
- In one partner's home, sometimes with a relative in the next room—a nerve-racking experience
- In one partner's home when no one is there, with a rushed feeling, listening for the sound of parents' footsteps—with a guilty sensation of sneaking around

Because of these experiences, some teenagers begin to associate sex with sleaziness. This is sad.

❖

What do girls feel after their first intercourse? Is it pure ecstasy? In one survey, more than half the girls questioned said they felt shame and worry.[7]

❖

For some girls, there is pain with the first intercourse. There can be pain with the tearing of the hymen, the connective tissue that partially closes across the vagina. And if the girl is fearful or quite stressed, she may experience powerful muscle contractions in the vagina, making intercourse extremely painful.

❖

Many sexually active teens are constantly fearful of pregnancy. How romantic can intercourse be when you're scared that you or your partner is getting pregnant?

Could sex be boring?

Lesley Jane Nonkin Seymour, who did a survey of teenage girls for a national teen magazine, says that few girls who are sexually active actually find sex physically satisfying. Many have never reached orgasm, and many report that while they continue to have sex with their boyfriends, they find sex boring.[8] At a young age, they've already had enough.

A common fantasy: to be a virgin again

A common fantasy of girls who have lost their virginity is to be a virgin again.

Boys experience "equipment failure"

Many boys fail completely in their first sexual intercourse. They experience "equipment failure"—an inability to achieve erection—that causes embarrassment and anxiety, as well as much worry about their sexual ability.

If a boy fails repeatedly, this can cause anxiety that continues into adulthood and can endanger future relationships.

❖

When you're a teenager, you've got more important things to worry about than the quality of your sexual performance.

Worries and pressures

Here are a few of the things teens experience in early intercourse:
- The boy may be impotent (unable to maintain an erection) due to fear
- Both partners are scared and anxious
- They don't use birth control and may conceive a baby
- They don't know how to do it
- The girl doesn't experience orgasm and feels little pleasure
- The two are too shy to communicate about what they are doing
- Sex is fumbling and unromantic, and the partners feel ashamed

❖

Teens may find themselves feeling guilty, confused, and anxious after deciding to have sex. Even young people who thought they had no hang-ups about sex can find themselves stressed and depressed. More than 80 percent of girls who have had sex wish they hadn't, according to one survey of U.S. teens.[9]

❖

One teen explains, "It's not like I planned to have sex. It just happened. Well maybe subconsciously I wanted it to happen. But it's not something I feel great about. Jackie and I aren't even together anymore. I feel sorry and let down about the whole thing. I thought sex would mean something. I thought I'd feel good about it."

❖

More girls than boys report that they had sex on a date even though they didn't really feel like it. This is especially true of girls sixteen and under. The younger the girl, the likelier she is to give in to sexual pressure.[10]

❖

Indiana University researchers found that teenage girls who are sexually active are more prone to sadness, sleeplessness, loneliness, school problems, and attempted suicide.[11]

❖

Studies show that when teenagers become sexually active, boys' grades fall and girls' desire to go to college is negatively affected.[12]

Guilt and teens

Shelly, a seventeen-year-old, says, "Most of my friends feel guilty after they have sex. . . . I don't think they're having much fun."[13]

❖

Teens who are raised in solidly middle-class homes may be surprised at the deep feelings of guilt that can accompany sexual activity.

❖

Twice as many girls as boys feel guilt and shame after their first sexual intercourse. Some girls feel so bad about what they've done that they require counseling to help them recover their self-esteem.

Feelings of guilt can eat away at you. Author Judith Viorst describes "that clutch in the stomach, that chill upon the soul, that self-inflicted misery called guilt. . . . If we breach [our] moral constraints or abandon [our] ideals, our conscience will observe, reproach, condemn . . . will arrange to make us feel guilty."[14]

WHY DO TEENS FEEL GUILTY ABOUT SEX?

Here are some big reasons why teenagers feel guilty about sex:

- **Religious reasons.** Teens who have been raised in a religion that teaches the immorality of premarital sex are especially likely to suffer from guilt after sexual activity.
- **Moral reasons.** It's been drilled into you throughout your life that premarital sex is immoral.
- **Your parents' teachings.** They've told you time after time that sex before marriage can screw up your life in lots of ways, and you know it's an incredibly big deal with them.
- **Cultural reasons.** Much of your culture is built on the ideal of marriage, monogamy (sex only with one's marriage partner), family, and commitment.

Sex with a sad twist

When you have sex and then suffer from guilt, as so many young people do, you are learning to associate something wonderful with feeling awful. It's a twisted way to begin the sexual side of your life. A surprising number of teens continue to carry these bad feelings about sex into adulthood. It can affect their future enjoyment of sex with their marriage partner. Marriage and sex counselors say this is a problem they deal with surprisingly often.

How can guilt cause pregnancy?

You may be surprised to learn that guilt is a leading cause of teen pregnancy. Because they feel guilty about sex, some teens "forget" to use birth control. They feel that if they were to come prepared (with a condom or other means of birth control), they would be admitting to themselves and their partner that the sex was planned. So, rather than plan ahead, they risk pregnancy by letting sex "just happen." They do this because they are trying to avoid a guilty conscience.

❖

Guilt can make us behave in destructive ways. Sometimes girls feel so guilty over having had a sexual relationship that, if they become pregnant, they view the pregnancy as a punishment for their behavior. Instead of giving their babies a better chance in life by placing them for adoption, they decide they must raise these children as punishment for their "sin." What a sad burden for a newborn to bear.

Sex can be joyous

Sex can indeed be joyous, but a joyful sexual relationship doesn't occur just because you have sex. It doesn't occur because you feel an intense attraction to another person. Shared sexual joy takes time.

❖

What is a good lover? Someone who can communicate well with their partner—someone who can talk, listen, and understand. Throughout your teenage years you will be perfecting your communication skills, but you will likely be around twenty before you are skilled enough to talk seriously with another person about what they like and dislike in many areas, including sex.

❖

Author Nancy Friday, who believes that postponing sexual activity is wise for young teens, states, "Sex does not make a woman of you. It is your reward for having made a woman of yourself first." [15] The same could be said for young men.

❖

When teens mature and marry, they begin to see that sex within a close, committed relationship is much more satisfying than casual sex, self-conscious sex, or sex without real trust. They learn to see sex as an intimate form of communication between two people who feel safe and relaxed in each other's arms. Most teen sex is a pale and painful version of this later intimacy.

chapter 5

Pregnancy:

It Could Happen to You

A teenage girl recalls, "I just couldn't talk to my boyfriend about birth control or condoms. I was way too embarrassed. It was okay for a while, but then I got pregnant. I couldn't believe it. I thought it could never happen to me."

Fifteen-year-old Jenn says, "Jamie and I had been going out for about a month. One night when his parents were away, we got a chance to be alone at his house. We were making out hot and heavy, and we just got completely carried away and did it. Jamie pulled out at the last second. He said everything would be okay and I couldn't get pregnant. But something must have gone wrong because I did. It was awful. I had an abortion. I thought Jamie loved me—at least, he acted like it before we did it. But after the abortion, he told me he didn't want to see me. Well, I don't ever want to have anything to do with him again."

Another teen explains, "I was brought up to believe that sex before marriage was wrong. But somehow Peter and I let things go too far. Sure, I was worried about getting pregnant. But I hated the thought of condoms, jellies, diaphragms and all that sick stuff. I knew I'd feel like a sleaze if I used birth control—like I planned the whole thing. And I didn't want Peter to think I was that kind of girl. So I didn't use protection. I don't know why I was so surprised when the doctor said I was pregnant."

"I'd never seen a condom before," said one young girl. "I'd heard about them, and I just figured he must be using one. No way was I going to ask him. We only had sex a couple of times—and I got pregnant."

A boy comments, "The baby's due in a couple of months, and I still don't know what to do. My girlfriend always seems depressed, and her mom and dad hate me. I know I'm responsible for all this mess, too, and I want to help her, but what can I do? We're too young to get married, and besides, I don't think we're exactly in love or anything anyway. I wish my life could be the way it was before all this happened. All I do is worry."

WHEN A MALE AND FEMALE HAVE SEX WITHOUT BIRTH CONTROL, NO ONE should be the least bit surprised if the girl becomes pregnant. The boy's sexual parts and the girl's sexual parts are designed to try their hardest to create a pregnancy *every* time intercourse occurs.

When a boy ejaculates into a girl's vagina, about 500 million sperm are released. They swim furiously toward the uterus. All it takes is for one sperm to unite with an egg in the fallopian tube and a baby will be created. Our reproductive parts were designed for success.

Teens tend to feel invulnerable. They have a sense that nothing bad will happen to them, even if they take risks. For example, many mistakenly believe, "If I have sex without protection, I won't get pregnant. I'm too young. I don't have sex that often. It's a safe time of the month. Nothing bad will happen to me."

Psychologist David Elkind calls this feeling of invulnerability a teenager's "personal fable"[1]—a feeling that bad things happen to *other people, not to them.* Unfortunately, this way of thinking leads to dangerous behavior.

The truth is that more than a million teenagers get pregnant every year. One out of five pregnancies begins in the very first month after a girl starts having sex.[2]

3,000 teens get pregnant every day!

More than 3,000 teenage girls get pregnant every day in the U.S. That's an average of one teenage pregnancy every thirty seconds, twenty-four hours a day. Many of these girls know about contraception (birth control methods), but they still don't use protection. They believe pregnancy just can't happen to them.

According to an eighteen-year-old teen mother named Laura, "When I looked at all the teen moms I was like, 'That's not going to happen to me . . . because I'm smarter than that.' I had things I wanted to do. . . . I had a whole bunch of dreams then. I started going out with [my boyfriend] when we were both fifteen. The first time I had sex with him I got pregnant. He was a virgin, and I had only had sex once before that. . . . I found out that I was pregnant, and it felt like it wasn't real." [3]

❖

Many mistakenly believe that teen pregnancy is a problem only among minority groups. The fact is, seven out of every ten teen births in the U.S. are to whites. [4]

Are you "too young" to get pregnant?

Young teens shouldn't think that they don't need birth control because they're "too young" to get pregnant. Kids their age get pregnant every day. Even ten-year-old girls can become pregnant.

❖

Even if a girl hardly ever has sex, she can get pregnant the one time she does. Some teens get pregnant the very first time.

❖

Even if you have friends who have unprotected sex and haven't gotten pregnant, they have just been lucky. Eventually they will get pregnant. Maybe next week.

❖

Susan, who is seven months pregnant, says, "We didn't use any kind of birth control. I know we should have. . . . We didn't think about this happening. We just did what we wanted. Our attitude was, 'Who cares?' We both had been with other people and it hadn't happened, even though neither of us used anything." [5]

How it happens

When a girl is about twelve, she begins having menstrual periods. When she is a little older, she begins to ovulate. About once a month, one of her ovaries releases an egg, which enters her fallopian tube. If the egg meets a sperm, it is fertilized and then travels to the uterus where it implants and develops into a baby. Fertilization usually occurs midway between menstrual cycles but has been known to occur at any time, even during menstruation. A girl's menstrual cycle can change unexpectedly at any time without her knowledge—meaning that there is NO guaranteed "safe" time for unprotected sexual intercourse. A pregnancy can occur unexpectedly unless birth control is used correctly EVERY TIME. Many teenagers—boys and girls—tend not to use birth control regularly. This is a simple fact.

❖

When sperm and egg unite, he becomes a father and she becomes a mother. Ready or not.

❖

If a girl hasn't started having her menstrual periods, she can still get pregnant. Ovulation (the release of an egg by an ovary) may occur about two weeks before a girl's first period, and at this time she could become pregnant.

There are NO safe days

The timing of ovulation can vary with illness and stress. And what teenager doesn't experience stress?

❖

Even the experts can't predict just when each girl will ovulate or when she will be most likely to conceive a baby.

❖

It is possible for a girl to ovulate more than once a month, according to sex educator and author Dr. James Leslie McCary. He explains that, during sexual excitement, even if it occurs during menstruation, an additional egg may be released.[6]

❖

Can a girl get pregnant if a boy uses the "withdrawal" method of birth control? Yes. (See page 56.) Even if the boy manages to withdraw his penis before he ejaculates (releases semen, which contains sperm), there will already be sperm in the pre-ejaculate fluid that oozes out in the minutes before withdrawal. These sperm immediately begin moving toward the egg to fertilize it.

Heavy petting and pregnancy

It is possible for a virgin to get pregnant during very heavy petting. If the tip of the penis gets anywhere near the vaginal opening, a pregnancy can occur. If sperm in the boy's semen happen to come in contact with the vagina, they can swim upward to the uterus and a baby can begin to grow.

❖

If sperm is released on the girl's leg or thigh, and if the boy or girl touches the sperm with a finger and then touches the vagina, a pregnancy is possible.[7]

❖

Douching (flooding the vaginal area with water or douching liquid) doesn't necessarily prevent pregnancy and sometimes even helps the sperm reach the uterus.

❖

After a boy ejaculates in the vagina, it only takes twenty seconds for sperm to reach the uterus.

❖

There is a 90 percent chance that a girl will get pregnant within a year if she has sex without birth control.[8]

❖

Most teens think pregnancy won't happen to them. Yet one out of three sexually active girls gets pregnant before the end of her teenage years.[9]

❖

If asked, most teens will say they believe in acting responsibly when it comes to birth control. Yet, in the heat of the moment, many do not.

❖

Many well-informed, middle-class and upper-class girls are among those who have sex without birth control.

WHAT YOU DON'T KNOW CAN HURT YOU

There is a lot of misinformation going around about how you prevent pregnancy. Below are only a few of the FALSE statements that naive girls have relied upon:

- If he withdraws, I can't get pregnant. (FALSE)
- If we do it standing up, I can't get pregnant. (FALSE)
- If I have irregular periods, I can't get pregnant. (FALSE)
- I can only get pregnant a couple of days each month. (FALSE)
- If I don't have an orgasm, I can't get pregnant. (FALSE)
- If I haven't started my periods yet, I can't get pregnant. (FALSE)
- If I only have sex once without protection, I can't get pregnant. (FALSE)
- I'm just a kid. I can't get pregnant. (FALSE)
- I have this very strong feeling that I won't get pregnant. I'm just sure I won't. (FALSE)

Birth Control

There is an amazing amount of information about birth control available to teens—more than ever before. Yet thousands of teenage girls get pregnant in the U.S. every day.

❖

After they begin to have sex, more than half of sexually active girls wait at least a year before seeking contraceptive services from a doctor or clinic. [10]

❖

Even when partners take measures to prevent pregnancy, they may fail. More than half of the women who have abortions say they were using contraception that failed. [11]

❖

Lorian Tonna, a nurse-counselor in Massachusetts, says that many of the girls she talks with are experiencing some type of abuse from their sex partners—hitting, slapping, rapes, or put-downs. "They might want to abstain or use birth control, but they don't because they are not in charge of their relationship," she explains. "Strange as it sounds, many of these girls harbor very romantic notions about their abusers."

She says, "There is tremendous pressure to have a relationship, any relationship. . . . They are willing to go along with the abuse . . . because they can't face the idea of not having a boyfriend." [12]

Guys may say pregnancy is the girl's fault

Many boys think birth control is a girl's responsibility. Consequently, some boys may know little or nothing about contraception, even though their girlfriends assume otherwise. Teens may be shy about talking to each other about birth control because they assume that others know more than they do and they don't want to look innocent or stupid.

❖

In one survey of teenage boys, half said it was the girl's fault if pregnancy occurred. If a girl gets pregnant, these boys would criticize her for not having "protected herself." [13]

❖

Unless both sexes understand their responsibility for birth control every time, pregnancy is probable.

❖

What's more important? Having sex for a few minutes or finishing high school and college, being free to develop great friendships, preparing for a job you'll enjoy, and having a nice place to live with a spouse and family you'll feel terrific about? Unprotected teenage sex puts all these things at risk.

WHY YOUNG PEOPLE DON'T USE BIRTH CONTROL

Here are a few reasons why teens who know about birth control don't use it when having sex:

- They don't think anything bad will happen.
- Girls think that if they use contraception or supply a boy with a condom, boys will think they planned to have sex. And they don't want to look like "that kind of a girl."
- Boys may be afraid to come prepared with condoms because they worry that the girl will think, "He must think I'm easy. He expected it."
- Many teens can't admit, even to themselves, that they are going to have sex, so they don't have any plan for contraception. They think of sex as something they could do only if they had an irresistible urge beyond their control.
- Both sexes are too guilty or embarrassed to buy condoms or to bring up the subject with their partners.
- Both sexes are too embarrassed or timid to bring up the subject of contraception with their doctor.
- Both sexes have a feeling that discussing contraception is unromantic, shameful, or disgusting.
- Both may think that condoms spoil the spontaneity of sex.

- Some boys insist that condoms interfere with sensitivity, and some girls are too embarrassed to argue.

- Some girls may say a condom is too irritating, and boys are too embarrassed to argue.

- Older guys dating younger girls may simply refuse to wear a condom. Young girls may not have the nerve to argue when an older boy says, "Don't worry about it. Nothing will happen. Go with the moment."

- Girls don't know how to respond when a boy says, "I've never been exposed to AIDS, so we don't need to use a condom. Anyway, I promise not to come inside you."

- Boys are afraid that if they stop long enough to put on a condom, the girl will change her mind.

- Boys may fear embarrassment if they can't apply a condom easily, so, rather than appear inexperienced, they skip the condom.

- Each partner assumes the other is using protection when neither is.

- Sex in movies and on TV never involves condoms. It looks romantic, and characters on TV rarely get diseases or have unwanted pregnancies. Teens see unprotected sex in the media, so they think maybe it's okay.

Can you imagine yourself falling into one of these traps? No one is immune.

What's the "withdrawal" method of birth control?

Many teens rely on withdrawal, or "coitus interruptus," for birth control. This means that the penis is withdrawn from the vagina just before ejaculation. Relying on withdrawal as a means of birth control is very risky. It calls for a boy to withdraw at the moment he has the greatest urge not to.

❖

This method is also a poor idea because the penis leaks sperm into the vagina before withdrawal.

❖

It is very easy for the boy to misjudge exactly when he should withdraw. If he misjudges, he may suddenly ejaculate into the vagina.

❖

A boy may be so excited that he just can't pull out in the middle of sex.

❖

Every year, 30 percent of the women relying on the withdrawal method will become pregnant. [14]

Some sobering statistics

Half of teen pregnancies occur within the first six months after a girl begins to have intercourse. [15]

❖

About 37,000 girls age fifteen and younger in the U.S. give birth in a given year. [16]

❖

Here's one that girls need to think hard about: Half the babies born to girls age fifteen to seventeen had fathers who were twenty years old or older. [17] Dating older boys or men may seem cool or be a status symbol, but it's taking an awful chance with your future. Older guys are much more likely to persuade younger girls to have sex, often without birth control or protection against STD (sexually transmitted disease).

How would pregnancy affect your relationship?

There's a good chance the boy will be angry with the girl for becoming pregnant or for failing to use contraceptives properly. She may hear, "Getting pregnant was your fault. It's your problem. You deal with it."

❖

"I dated John for about a year," says Robyn. "He always told me that if anything happened he would take care of me. When I told him I was pregnant he said that it wasn't his baby. He dropped me and started dating my best friend. It was hard for me to accept that he didn't care as much as he said he did before I got pregnant." [18]

❖

When a girl becomes pregnant her boyfriend may insist, "The baby must be someone else's." But court-ordered paternity tests can prove otherwise.

❖

Nine out of ten boys abandon their pregnant girlfriends. Some may have had strong feelings for the girl, but they are just not mature enough to handle something this big.

❖

Getting pregnant and having a baby are not the way to get or keep a man.

❖

When a girl gets pregnant, she may see what she thought was a deep, romantic relationship explode in her face. If she and her partner had kept sex out of it, they might have hung on to something special.

How does pregnancy affect a girl's life?

"Pregnancy in unmarried teenagers is a disaster for everyone involved. . . . These pregnancies result in sadness and heartbreak, not only for the girl and boy involved, but for their families and for the infant," says Dr. Wilson W. Grant, a sex educator. [19]

❖

Because the teenage father usually wants nothing more to do with her, the girl is left alone to deal with the agonizing decisions about abortion, adoption, or raising the baby.

❖

57

Faced with telling their parents about an unwanted pregnancy, teens are often confused about what to do. Some run away, some secretly have abortions, and some attempt suicide. For most teens, the wisest thing to do is to tell their parents immediately and trust in their help and advice.

❖

Pregnant teenage girls are seven times as likely to commit suicide as other girls.

❖

The pregnant teenager may put off telling her parents for months. She may be paralyzed by anxiety, shame, and guilt. She may have difficulty concentrating, problems sleeping, no appetite, or she may "be in a frenzy of compulsive overeating." [20]

❖

Teen pregnancy is the leading reason why girls drop out of school. It is thought to be the leading reason for boys as well. A third of teen mothers drop out of school. [21]

❖

Teen pregnancy often contributes to a lifelong cycle of poverty.

What do pregnant teens face at school?

The pregnant teen at school may be an object of gossip, stares, and whispers.

❖

A pregnant teen named Katy said she felt a "coolness" from the other kids at school. "I was kind of set aside. It bothered me, but I tried not to let it." [22]

❖

"Going to school while I was pregnant was . . . hard," says Sarah. "The whispers, the looks. . . . People I thought I could depend on turned their backs on me. Even some of my teachers were biased against me because I was pregnant." [23]

❖

Another teen who got pregnant at fifteen recalls, "I didn't tell any of my friends because we always talked about going to the same college, seeing the world, and never talked about kids. I was embarrassed to bring it up. I didn't know what they would think about me. They would think it was cute for a while, but their parents would look at me like a slut and tell them not to hang around with me. I ended up dropping out of school, not wanting anybody to see me pregnant." [24]

What does the boy go through?

When a teenage boy finds out that he is going to be a father, he may need counseling to deal with his fear, guilt, confusion, and grief. He may feel that his life is falling apart.

❖

While most boys want nothing more to do with their pregnant girl-friends, a few do want to participate in decisions regarding the pregnancy. In many cases, the girl's parents won't let them, and they may be ignored by social service agencies. [25]

❖

In a teen magazine, a nineteen-year-old boy wrote about how he felt when his girlfriend told him she was pregnant. "I was sick with stress. As the father, I had no say. What I wanted didn't matter and what I felt was of no consequence. Sure, Katie was worried about me and my feelings, but ultimately the decision was hers. It's her body. Not mine. That was the most frustrating thing. I felt like, 'It's not my body, but it's my life.' I felt responsible for the whole thing, yet I felt completely powerless. It wasn't fair. The choice [not to have an abortion] was final and I had to live with it." [26]

❖

When teen fathers are pushed out of the scene, they may give up try-ing to support their pregnant partner and, later, their child. Society makes them feel like they've screwed up. The mother and child may be scooped up by a social service agency, while the father is locked out, confused, and frightened, and left feeling bad about himself. [27]

There are serious effects on a girl's health

Pregnant teens are more likely to suffer medical complications from pregnancy and childbirth than older mothers. These compli-cations include long labor, high blood pressure, and anemia.

❖

Because girls do not typically reach full height until four or five years after they first have periods, it is possible for pregnancy to stunt the young mother's growth.[28] This means she may not grow as tall as she otherwise could have.

❖

One out of three pregnant teens doesn't receive adequate prenatal care (the very important medical care during the nine months before childbirth).[29] Pregnant teens have higher rates of toxemia, miscarriage, birth complications, and maternal death than older women who become pregnant.

❖

The risk of death for sixteen- to nineteen-year-olds who give birth is 13 percent higher than for women in their twenties.[30]

❖

Although young teens are able to become pregnant, their bodies aren't yet mature enough to give the developing baby the best possible chance. The bones of the pelvic girdle are still growing and do not reach full size until a girl is older.[31] Thus, the baby's head may be too large to fit through the birth canal, causing a long, difficult, and excessively painful labor that puts mother and child at risk.

What about the health of the baby?

Does the decision to have sex involve only the teen and their partner? What about the other potential person in this event—the baby? Teen sexual activity can risk the health and well-being of an innocent third person.

❖

"No one ever told me that my child's life might end . . . before he could take his first breath," a teenager writes to advice columnist Ann Landers. She and her boyfriend had just chosen a headstone and made funeral arrangements for their infant. "I am now going through something no teenager should ever have to face. And they are right—my life will never be the same."[32]

Teenage girls sometimes have such difficulty facing the reality of pregnancy that they deny the pregnancy, even to themselves. If they continue smoking, drinking, abusing drugs, or using some prescription medications (even for acne or seizures), they are putting their baby's health at serious risk.

❖

New studies show that, even with adequate prenatal care, teens are more likely to have low birth-weight infants and to deliver prematurely. [33] This means the baby is born too soon and does not have enough time inside the mother to develop completely. Its organs may not be fully formed, and this can lead to breathing problems and bleeding in the brain. Low birth-weight babies are forty times more likely to die during their first few weeks of life as babies of normal weight. [34]

❖

Babies of teen mothers are at greater risk of birth defects, birth injuries, blindness, deafness, cerebral palsy, motor problems, epilepsy, mental retardation, and other problems.

❖

Have you ever felt angry and hurt because you thought your parents mistreated you? By having sex as a teen, are you at risk of mistreating your potential child?

chapter 6

....

LISTEN UP, GUYS!

Eighteen years of child support is a long time!

"A baby costs $474 a month. How much do you have in your pocket?" asks attorney Anne Browning Wilson to a group of high school students. "I have heard judges say nearly these same words many times in court. Young fathers come to court for the first time to be ordered to pay child support, and when they find out they will be making large payments each month for years, until they are middle-aged, they are devastated.

"I agree with the child support laws, but I feel sorry for these boys. Why didn't anyone tell them about these laws before, back when it would have mattered? When they could have done things differently and avoided this disaster to their lives? Why weren't child support laws taught in their sex education classes?" [1]

SOME TEENS SAY, "IF IT FEELS GOOD, DO IT." "I'M NOT HURTING ANYBODY." "Hey, I'm young—this is my chance to live a little." "My girlfriend says it's okay, so it's nobody's business but ours."

These young people may not have given much thought to how easily an unplanned pregnancy can occur. And it appears that they know nothing about their state's child support laws.

What do you know about child support? What you don't know might just blow you away. If a teenage boy gets his girlfriend pregnant, he is legally obligated to help support their baby until the child is eighteen, even if he never marries the girl or ever sees her or the baby again. This means he must send large payments every month to his former girlfriend until he is thirty-five to forty years

63

old! Even if the unwed father marries someone else, has other children, and needs all his money for his new family, he must continue to support his out-of-wedlock child. This means that he and his current family may have to do without many of the things they would enjoy having, maybe even things they seriously need.

If a young man paying child support to his former girlfriend meets a woman he wants to marry, this new love may hesitate or back out of the relationship. She may view eighteen years of his paying child support (even longer if he supports his child in college) as just too great a financial burden on their marriage.

All fifty states have child support laws. A teen father is required to pay child support even if he is a "child" himself and has no job. Fathers as young as fourteen have been required by the courts to pay child support. A boy suddenly responsible for eighteen years of child support payments may see his dreams and plans for life go up in smoke.

The following are some commonly asked questions about child support from a brochure called "If We Make a Baby, Do I Have to Pay?" written by attorney Anne Browning Wilson.[2]

Q. My sex partner and I had a baby. We've decided not to marry or live together, and my sex partner is going to keep and raise the child. Do I have to pay to help support our child?

A. YES! We have laws requiring both parents to share the costs of raising their child until the child is eighteen years old. This means that if you are the parent without custody, you will be making monthly payments to the court until you are middle-aged, even if you would rather spend that money on a home, car, clothes, food, other bills, or a little fun. It is a high price to pay for being careless when you were younger, but it's the law.

Q. Why do we have "child support laws"?

A. They are not designed to punish you, but to make sure that all children have decent lives. Your child should not have to live in poverty just because he or she lives with only one parent.

We also have laws that give you the opportunity to take an active role in raising your child even if you do not have custody.

Q. How can the court prove who the real father is?

A. Modern blood and genetic tests can prove if a particular person is the father. The court can require him to participate in these expensive tests (costing more than $600) and can make him pay for them if he is found to be the father. These tests will also quickly prove he is not the father if he has been wrongfully named.

Knowing who both parents are is important because children need the friendship and love of both a mother and father. Sometimes the child needs to know for medical reasons.

Q. What if the father wants his girlfriend to have an abortion or put the child up for adoption and she refuses?

A. He must still pay to support the child. He has no legal right to force her to have an abortion or give up the baby for adoption.

Q. How much will I have to pay for child support?

A. The judge adds together the incomes of both parents and checks a chart that sets child support amounts according to the parents' total income. Basically, the higher this total income is, the higher the child support amount will be. You will also help pay birth expenses, including doctors, hospital, etc.

Example: If the father earns twice as much as the mother who has custody, he will pay two-thirds of the support amount.

Example: If a mother earns the same amount as the father who has custody, she will pay one-half the support amount.

The parent with custody is considered to have paid his or her share by paying many of the expenses for the child who lives in the home.

Q. How much will it cost in all, over the entire eighteen years?

A. Families with one child spend about one-fourth of their income on that child. The total child support amount for one child could range anywhere from around $50,000 to $250,000, depending on the income of the parents.

Q.What if I'm still in high school and only have a part-time job?

A. Each case is different, but the court may have you pay a minimum amount while you are in high school and increase it when you get out and get a full-time job. In the meantime, your partner may have to go on welfare, and you may have to pay back some of the taxpayers' money when you get a job.

Q. What if I planned to go to college before working full-time? Will the judge let me keep paying this low amount until I finish college?

A. Again, every case is different, but probably not. It's nice that you wanted to go to college, but the judge will probably point out that your partner may have wanted to go to college, too. Instead, he or she has a full-time job as a parent and needs your financial help to raise the baby right now—not in four years.

You will probably have to work full-time to make your child support payment, and try to go to college part-time through night classes, if you have enough energy after working all day.

Q. I know of a father who doesn't pay any child support. If I refuse, how can they MAKE me pay?

A. It used to be common for parents without custody to try to avoid payment. However, new laws make it very difficult to avoid paying. If you miss one of your monthly payments, the court can:

- Make your boss pay money from your wages directly to the court
- Take over your bank accounts
- Make you sell your property
- Put you in jail

Q. If I leave the state, can they still make me pay?

A. Yes. There is a law that requires courts in one state to collect child support for courts in other states.

Q. If the parent with custody has never asked me for money and goes on welfare, then I'm off the hook, right?

A. Wrong. In this case, the parent with custody is required to name you—the other parent. Then you will be located by one of the state's team of lawyers whose special job is to track down parents without custody and make them pay.

Q. If the parent with custody marries, does the new step-parent take over support, so that I don't have to pay anymore?

A. No. A step-parent has no legal duty to support a step-child. Only if someone legally adopts your child does your duty to pay support end. If you want to avoid eighteen years of child support payments, and would rather spend your money on your own needs and wants, or on a spouse and children you choose to have, then you must avoid an unplanned pregnancy.

Your career could come to a screeching halt

"Deadbeat Dads," those who don't pay their child support, also risk the loss of their income tax refunds and their professional license (a license that allows them to work as a plumber, doctor, truck driver, builder, or other licensed professional). In other words, their careers are over—unless they pay up. Likewise, they will be denied government loans for a home, business, or farm unless they pay their child support.

❖

An increasing number of states are suspending the driver's licenses of men and women who don't pay their child support. Imagine trying to make it in life without being allowed to drive a car.

❖

The goal, said President Bill Clinton of efforts to enforce child support, is to let fathers know that "we're not going to just let you walk away from your children and stick the taxpayers with the tab. We have to make responsibility a way of life, not an option."[3]

❖

New welfare reform laws cut off payments to moms who refuse to name their baby's father. Even if the father isn't named until years after the birth, he may be required to pay back the taxpayers' money that his partner got from the government.

❖

In one recent case, a father was suddenly required to pay $60,000 in back child support for a son he never knew he had.

❖

You may have seen FBI "Ten Most Wanted" posters of criminals on the bulletin board at your local post office. Now the government is displaying similar posters of photos of deadbeat parents with their names, occupations, and last known addresses.

❖

Teenage girls should not get the impression that if they have a baby, the child support laws will mean that they will be taken care of. Enforcement is getting better, but still only about half of court-ordered child support gets paid. "Many desperately poor teenage moms are in the half that gets nothing," says attorney Wilson.[4]

....

chapter 7

Difficult Choices:

Options for the pregnant teen and her partner

A young man describes how he felt when his girlfriend told him she was pregnant: "I was in shock. . . . I felt like I lost it—like I lost everything. . . . After she dropped the bomb that night, my head kept screaming, 'What are we going to do?' The answer was always the same: I wanted this whole thing to just go away. The more I thought about it, the more I started to believe that my solution was the only solution: I wanted her to have an abortion—for a lot of reasons." [1]

Christina, seventeen, who decided to put her baby up for adoption: "I know I can't keep my baby. I can't give it all the things a baby needs and I sure can't dump it on my parents because they can't afford to take care of their own family. I've decided to give it up for adoption. I think it's better for the baby to give it up to parents who can't have a baby for themselves. I think that I'm really doing a favor to my baby, although I'm always going to wonder what it looks like and what it's doing." [2]

A teen who's raising her baby: "I got pregnant a year and a half ago. My best friend talked to me a lot about getting an abortion, but I just couldn't go through with it. I decided to have the baby and let him be adopted. But after he was born, I couldn't part with him. I felt this rush of love, like I knew he depended on me to be his mother. But I wasn't ready for how things would be. I'm just so tired all the time. The diapers, the laundry, the sickness, the crying. I never get a good night's sleep. It's such hard work. Sometimes I think I'm gonna explode. I don't like to admit it cause I do love my baby, but there are these times when I think I hate him too."

The teenage mother of a one-year-old complains, "I've had enough. I never get to go shopping or see my friends. It's like my life is over. I'm only sixteen, and I already ruined everything."

ABORTION, ADOPTION, MARRIAGE, PARENTHOOD. LET'S SAY YOU (OR YOUR girlfriend) got pregnant. Which of these options would you choose? Does any one of them seem like a choice you could live with?

If you've ever thought to yourself, "If I/my girlfriend got pregnant, I'd just____," then keep reading for a closer look at the reality of each choice. None of these choices insures happiness, and some could bring permanent heartache. All can be avoided by postponing sex until you're a lot older and more mature.

Abortion

In recent decades, "abortion" has referred to a surgical procedure to remove the lining of the uterus, including the developing embryo or fetus. Abortion is legal in all fifty states. In 1997, the U.S. began clinical trials of drugs that induce abortion without surgery. Drug-induced abortions occur over a matter of one or more days.

❖

Teens who think of abortion as a means of "birth control" are irresponsible and ignorant. Abortion is far more expensive than contraception, and even teens who are pro-choice (believe abortion should be legally available) may suffer depression after the procedure. Furthermore, repeated abortions may cause long-term medical complications.

❖

If you get pregnant, do you "just go out and get an abortion," and all your problems are solved? Hardly.

❖

When a girl and boy decide on abortion, there is often much guilt and sadness. When it actually comes down to having an abortion, both partners may feel awful. It can be a heart-wrenching decision, one they may think about and struggle with for the rest of their lives.

❖

Teens who believe that abortion is wrong or that it ends a developing human life should think very hard about whether teen sexual activity is wise or fair. One out of three sexually active girls gets pregnant by the end of her teenage years. More than a third of teen pregnancies end in abortion.

❖

Hundreds of thousands of pregnant teenagers choose abortion, but not all teens who choose abortion can get one.

❖

Many states require that a girl get her parents' consent, or a judge's approval, before an abortion. Ideally, pregnant teens should be able to tell their parents about their predicament and look to their parents for help and understanding. For girls from stable, supportive homes, asking parents to consent to an abortion is very upsetting for everyone, but possible. But for girls who come from angry or troubled homes, talking with parents about their pregnancy can cause an explosive situation. Some girls are physically abused by angry parents.

❖

Sometimes girls with the best relationships with their families have the most awful time telling parents about their plans to obtain an abortion. Author-columnist and social commentator Anna Quindlen writes of these "girls who wanted their parents to have certain illusions about them . . . girls who wanted to remain good girls in the minds that mattered to them most."[3]

For some girls, it is unbearable to disappoint those who have loved, trusted, and cherished them the most. Rather than tell their parents, some risk illegal, secret abortions.

❖

The alternative to parent notification and consent is to request special permission from the court for a confidential abortion without parental involvement. Such a court hearing is no picnic. With judge, attorneys, and court personnel listening, a teenager must reveal deeply personal information about herself and her situation.

❖

Surgical abortions cost between $400 and $700. Drug-induced abortions are around $350. Few teens have this much money.

How boys may feel about the abortion

In some cases, the teenage father mourns the loss of the baby more than the mother, who may be very relieved to have the whole thing over with.

❖

If the boy comes from a family with strong anti-abortion feelings or has these feelings himself, he and his family may try legal options to prevent the abortion.

❖

On the other hand, many boys push their pregnant girlfriends to have an abortion because they do not wish to pay child support for eighteen years (see chapter 6). They do not want to be forced into a long relationship with the girl, whom they may no longer care for.

Girls still suffer from illegal, botched abortions

Of the thousands of teens who are unable to obtain legal abortions, most give birth to their babies. But some seek illegal abortions. Some become infected and die. Some are never again able to become pregnant.

❖

Some desperate girls attempt to abort the fetus themselves, using knitting needles or coat hangers in an often fatal attempt to remove the fetus. Others try vacuum cleaner suction, not realizing that this can make a hole in their uterus and suck in their intestines, causing death.[4]

❖

If a girl becomes pregnant and is unable to get an abortion, she should NEVER try to do the abortion herself and NEVER seek an abortion from someone unlicensed to perform one. It is usually best if she brings her parents in on her decision.

Adoption

If a girl thinks abortion is wrong and if she wants her baby to have a better life than she can offer, or if she has waited too long in her pregnancy to get an abortion, she may decide to go through with the pregnancy and put the baby up for adoption. Every year, thousands of pregnant teens realize they are too young to raise a baby. These young men and women offer their infants for adoption by older couples who desperately want a child to bring up in a home that is loving, stable, and financially secure. For many teens, the knowledge that they have "done the right thing" is bittersweet.

❖

Angelique, eighteen, decided during her pregnancy that she would let her baby be adopted. She recalls, "After the baby was born, it was hard for me to distance myself emotionally from [her]. I'm not even sure how I did it. . . . I cried for about four months nonstop." But in the end, Angelique says, she knew she made the right decision.[5]

❖

Before their twelve-day-old daughter Nora was given to adoptive parents, Andy and his girlfriend held and cared for the infant. Andy recalls, "It was so completely sad. I was a father but I didn't feel like one." About the adoption, he says that he and his girlfriend "were terrified that we were making a horrible mistake. But ultimately, we knew we had to go through with it—more for Nora than ourselves. . . . Since then the pain has not gone away."

Andy knows his daughter is in good hands, but laments, "I'm still trying to figure out who I am and who I was. I can't remember what it feels like not to worry, not to have the weight of the world on my shoulders."[6]

Some teens change their minds

Some teenage girls, who had every intention of allowing their babies to be adopted, change their minds. Experts believe that hormones circulating in the girl's body before and following the baby's birth trigger a strong "maternal instinct," an overpowering desire to care for the infant. So a girl's original decision to place her baby in a secure and stable home may be discarded in favor of a decision to try to raise the baby herself.

❖

Some pregnant teens are pressured by their friends to keep the baby. They don't realize that their friends' early fascination with the baby may soon disappear, and they will be left alone with the infant.

❖

The decision to put the baby up for adoption can give a teen mother and father the security of knowing that their baby will be raised in a good, loving home. Yet, when the child is gone, both may feel empty and forever curious about their child.

❖

It can be a very sad event for a teenage boy when his sex partner puts their newborn up for adoption if he does not want her to. Some boys take their partners to court to block the adoption.

❖

In recent years the courts have increasingly recognized an unmarried father's rights when it comes to adoption. The court may allow the teenage father to come up with his own plan for raising the child, and the teen mother may be ordered to pay child support for eighteen years.

Adoption later on can be a poor idea

Sometimes, after going through two or three years of raising their babies, teens decide that they just can't handle the situation any longer. They can't face the crying, clinging, dirty diapers, exhaustion, lack of social life, and poverty any longer. So they decide to place their toddlers for adoption. This may solve the teen's problems, but it causes the child terrible distress to lose its mother or father. And the older the child is, the harder it is to find an adoptive family. Most couples seek infants.

❖

Teens should understand that adoption can be a very complicated and difficult experience for all these reasons.

Is marrying each other going to fix things?

If you and your teen partner like each other very much, maybe even love each other, and, through carelessness, conceive a baby, is marriage a good idea? A good, solid marriage does not begin as a convenient solution to a problem. A good marriage occurs when two people have made a thoughtful decision to share each other's lives and to respect each other's views about things like finances, religion, a home, children, housework, leisure time, and careers.

❖

The life of married teenagers can be a life of great loneliness. They no longer have a place among their unmarried, dating friends. They share little in common with older married couples. The teen wife especially is confined by the baby's schedule and needs. Both partners suffer from a serious lack of money for outings. Even when they can go out, where can they go with a baby?[7] Sitters are expensive!

❖

Many married teen parents find themselves on welfare, food stamps, and other government aid programs. They slide quickly into debt and end up borrowing money at high interest rates just to make ends meet. Such poverty and indebtedness can put terrible stress on the marriage.

Where did the good times go?

What can you and your partner expect if you marry because of an unwanted pregnancy? To pay rent, buy food, pay doctor bills, and meet other expenses, both of you will need to get jobs. (Renting an unfurnished apartment can easily cost $500 a month. Other expenses may add an additional $1000 or more.) Your child will also need daycare, which can be quite expensive as well as a great worry. You will both be trying to complete high school and/or college and, of course, doing homework. Caring for the baby will consume the rest of your time and energy.

And don't forget saving money instead of having fun with it, paying bills, cleaning house, shopping for the basics, and doing boring errands and chores. You and your spouse may feel that you almost never see each other—let alone have a good time together. And if either of you drops out of school, you will be hurting your future chances at a good career and a better life.

❖

Teen mothers who marry are likely to drop out of school and never go back. They're more apt to join the work force at a younger age, have a less satisfying job, and earn less money than women who postpone motherhood and marriage.

❖

Boys who marry as teenagers are likely to have fewer skills, make less money, be fired more often, and have less chance for promotion.

❖

In general, teens who marry as a result of a pregnancy are more likely to get less education and to be stuck in lives of poverty.

Friendship and sex

At least if you're married, you'll always find comfort and friendship in your partner—right? Not necessarily. A teen wife may be exhausted by caring for a baby and other duties. She may hate being stuck at home day after day. A teen husband may resent his boring job and the end of his youth and freedom. He may feel a slow-burning anger toward his bride for having become pregnant in the first place. Each partner may blame the other for their miserable situation and broken dreams.

❖

But at least you'll finally have unlimited sex—right? Maybe not. Once you and your teen partner marry and take on the responsibilities of raising a child and making a living, you may both feel so troubled that you no longer find sex attractive. And, like many other teens, you may not have figured out much about each other's sexuality to begin with. The young husband doesn't know his wife's sexual needs and may be too upset most of the time to work things out with her. For her, sex may be unsatisfying and increasingly less interesting. Meeting with this lack of response, the teenage husband may feel frustrated and cheated.

"I hate my life"

A teenage wife writes to Ann Landers: "I hate my life. . . . The baby cries all the time and gets on Ted's nerves. He drinks too much and I can't blame him. We live in a dump and there is no money for sitters or movies or decent clothes. Ted never says anything but I know he must hate me. . . . I'm afraid he hates the baby, too. He never holds her or pays attention to her.

"There are times when I think this is all a bad dream and I'll wake up at home in my own bed, and get dressed and go to school with the kids I liked so much. But I know too well that those days are over for me and I am stuck. . . ."[8]

Reality hits hard

Of course, there are teen marriages that succeed. But to make things work out long term, partners must be mature, highly compatible, and focused on success. Many teens think their marriage will be the one great love that can overcome all obstacles, even though most others fail. Yet these teens face the same harsh problems as others, and when reality hits, it hits hard.

❖

A girl may feel especially hurt and angry when her husband continues to run around with the guys at night while she's stuck at home caring for the baby. He figures, "Why should both of us be tied down?" She feels left out and lonely.

❖

The two may discover before long that they really don't get along that well. They are not compatible. They just don't make a good husband-and-wife team. Their chance to date over a long period and get to know their differences was cut short by sex and pregnancy.

❖

Teen marriages often end in disaster. The teen divorce rate is twice as high as that of older couples.[9] When the marriage breaks up, the mother and baby are usually left struggling alone.

Parents need to feel good about themselves

When teens give birth to an out-of-wedlock child, chances are good that some people in their families will be ashamed of them and angry at them. This harsh treatment harms a girl's already shaky self-image. Whether we like it or not, we are all deeply affected by the opinions of those close to us, explains psychologist David Elkind.[10] He quotes a letter to Ann Landers in which the father of a teen mother says that his daughter has "denied me the joy of walking her down the aisle and giving her in marriage to a decent man I could be proud of. . . . Our daughter is a tramp."[11]

Most teenage girls couldn't help being emotionally damaged by such a cruel response from their fathers.

❖

Elkind says the best mother is one who has a healthy, strong self-image and high self-esteem. An older, married mom is more likely to feel better about who she is and what her place is in the world. A teenage mother is apt to be caught in an anxious marriage, struggling to make ends meet and care for a child. She is much less likely to feel good about herself and find satisfaction in child rearing. [12]

❖

Teenage years are a time when you're deeply involved in your own "identity crisis"—that is, figuring out who you are. Psychologists say that only when humans are older are they able to care deeply about the needs and hurts of others. Teens have so much personal growing still to do that it is difficult for them to nurture another person full-time.

How it is for the teen mother

What's it like to be a teen mother? Is it anything like the responsibility you have when you baby-sit for a few hours? There is no comparison. Teen motherhood is eighteen or more years' worth of nonstop, twenty-four-hour-a-day, hard work, worry, heavy responsibility, and agonizing emotional involvement. Teen moms find themselves short on good parenting skills and exhausted by their responsibilities.

❖

Because their lives are frustrating, many teen mothers are irritable and intolerant of annoying baby behaviors. Some are fed up with life in general and quickly lose their temper with their babies.

❖

When a teenager leaves her own childhood behind to raise a child, she may have a youth not of fun and freedom, but of stress and disillusionment. She may ask herself, "Why isn't this experience as beautiful as I imagined it would be? Why am I so tired all the time? Why does my baby cry so much?"

How it is for the teen father

Many teen fathers begin to lose interest in being fathers. They are just too stressed and overworked. They are not mature enough to handle so many problems. The children of most teen parents eventually end up with no father in the home.

How it is for the baby

A baby needs to be welcomed into the world by two mature and sensible parents.

❖

It really hurts to be a child whose father has left the scene or cares little about them.

❖

Having an involved father in the home is vital to a child's emotional well-being. Without a daddy, children's mental health and academic success suffer, according to David Popenoe in *Life Without Father*.[13] "Daddies matter, big time," says political strategist James Carville, outlining national social priorities for the U.S.[14]

Most girls raise the baby alone

Even though "daddies matter, big time," 90 percent of teenage fathers abandon their pregnant girlfriends. Hundreds of thousands of teenage girls raise their babies alone. What happens to the pregnant girl who raises her baby by herself?

- Does she move to a pretty, cozy apartment where she and her adorable, cuddly baby live in quiet happiness?
- Does the baby's love make her feel complete and fill her days with joy?
- Does the baby's father visit her often, providing affection, financial support, and attention?
- Does the teenage mom hire baby-sitters and resume her social life?
- Does she finish high school with her friends?
- Does she begin a meaningful career?

- Do her friends visit often, envy her independence, and think her baby is wonderful?

In most cases, the answer to all these questions is, NO.

❖

"I have been dating this guy for a while now," says a teen named Gwen, "and he and I have a three-year-old little girl together. I love him a lot and want to be with him all the time, but it seems that any chance I get to spend with him, he has something else going on."

❖

Most single teenage mothers live a life of poverty, ignored by old friends, abandoned by the baby's father, exhausted by the burden of child rearing with no husband to help out, and stuck in dead-end jobs or on welfare.

❖

Diane, a teen mom disappointed in her ex-boyfriend, says she expected him to be more committed to being a father. She says she expected him to say, "I'm going to help you. I'll be there to take care of Jimmy when you want, when you need to do other things." Diane explains, "I expected his support emotionally, financially, as much as he could. I expected him to be there for me . . . I expected him to love me because I was the woman who had his baby. But he loves everyone else who didn't." [15]

❖

Lisa, fifteen, relates, "Before I had the baby I was free. I had a lot of friends. I was fun to be with. I was happy. I enjoyed a lot of things, and I am just different now. I'm lonely. I'm quiet. I am not like I was anymore. I have changed completely."

Psychologist Carol Gilligan writes about Lisa in her book *In a Different Voice*. Lisa is confused and sad. Her boyfriend has left her, but she is still in love with him. Gilligan writes, "She is unable to see how an act of love can have led to such desolation and loss." [16]

Hoping for marriage to somebody — anybody

If a teenage mother doesn't marry the boy who fathered her baby, she is likely to marry a guy she might not otherwise have chosen. [17] This is because she is poor and alone and desperate. She hopes that marriage to somebody—even a partner who is less than ideal—will improve her life. Many teen moms never marry.

❖

When a girl becomes a teen mother, she loses her chance to decide what happens in her life. By postponing sex, she'll be assured of having time to finish her education, find a good job, meet a guy she really gets along with, and have a baby when the time is right for her and her husband.

How would the two of you manage?

A young girl is more likely than an older mother to give birth to a disabled child. (See "What about the health of the baby?" on page 60.) How would she and her boyfriend handle raising a child who is mentally retarded or has serious physical disabilities? Even mature adult couples are overwhelmed by this responsibility.

How do teen parents treat their babies?

Some teen parents do a remarkably good job of raising their child in spite of difficult obstacles. But some reject the child as if the child were the cause of all their troubles. Others smother their child with attention as a way to work off the guilt they feel over having brought the child into a troubled situation. Some are quick to punish and are not patient with the infant's normal, but annoying, behaviors.

❖

Teenage mothers have a higher rate of child abuse than older mothers. Even if they do not abuse their children physically, they may be more neglectful and may not give their kids enough protection and attention. [18] Their children are more likely to suffer physical, emotional, and social problems. [19]

Shaken baby syndrome

It's 5:30 P.M. You're trying to make dinner. The baby is crying, and you can't quiet him. The peas are burning. The TV is blaring. The dog is barking. You're late with the rent. And that awful screaming won't stop. You lose it totally. Your emotions go haywire, and you glare at the pudgy, red-faced, yowling little object of your frustration, grab his tiny shoulders, and shake the heck out of him—maybe that will shut him up! Hours later at the emergency room, they tell you you've damaged his brain. Your whole world dissolves.

"Shaken baby syndrome" has been much in the news in recent years. Angry, impatient, frustrated parents may try to shake their crying infants into silence, little knowing they are causing permanent harm. Pediatricians' offices feel compelled to put up notices in waiting areas warning about the dangers of this form of "punishment," which can result in tragic injury and criminal prosecution.

❖

In the city of Merrimack, New Hampshire, eighteen-year-old Robin Peters raised money for a project to make teens more aware of the difficulty of caring for an infant. Working at her family's doughnut shop, Robin earned money to buy three, $275 computerized "Baby Think It Over" dolls for the local high school.

The dolls are assigned to individual students for forty-eight hours to fulfill class requirements. The dolls cry loudly for random twenty-minute intervals day and night, stopping only when a key is inserted and held at the correct angle. An internal computer records if the doll was "abused" by shaking, dropping, or hitting. Students reach a point where they can't take it anymore, a teacher reports.

Robin decided to buy the dolls in memory of her own daughter, Amanda, who, at age six weeks, was shaken to death by the child's father. He is now in prison.[20]

❖

Being a parent is difficult at any age. Without a doubt, it is extremely difficult for teenage mothers and fathers to suddenly become parents while they are still children, themselves in need of nurturing and a chance to grow up.

The whole thing falls into Grandma's lap

Some teen mothers just give up and leave the scene. Often the baby's grandmother is left to care for the child, putting a terrible strain on the older woman's life.

"I just couldn't handle it anymore, so my mom's raising Kimmie back home," says eighteen-year-old Angie, who left the small Ohio town where she grew up. "It's hard for me to admit, even to myself, but after I left, Kimmie busted up Mom's marriage to my stepfather. He just couldn't take having a baby around. Now my mother works in a liquor store to get by, and Kimmie spends most of her day at the store with Mom. I know it's a weird place to bring up a little kid. Sometimes I can hardly stand how guilty I feel about everything."

What happens when these babies grow up?

Children of teen parents have a rough life in many ways. Compared to children of older parents, they tend to have poorer growth, more problems in school, reading difficulties, lower IQs, lower grades, and problems with drug use. They tend to repeat their parents' lives by getting pregnant younger, marrying younger, having poor parenting skills, and divorcing more often.

When teens postpone sex until they're older, they help break this vicious cycle of hundreds of thousands of unplanned babies, who grow up to have more unplanned babies, and so on. Doesn't every baby deserve the love and good parenting skills of a mature couple? By postponing sex, you are giving your future little ones the best chance at a good life.

chapter 8

·····················

Is Everybody Doing It?

Peer pressure and self-esteem

Trish, age sixteen, reflects, "I felt dirty, I really felt dirty. I felt that I had deceived my mother in a way, too, because she had always told me, 'Wait till you're sure, wait till you're sure.' And I wasn't sure. I just did it because everyone else was doing it. And it didn't feel good, and I didn't like it, and I thought it sucked all around." [1]

A young woman explains, "All of my friends were doing it and they dared me. After all, I was seventeen and had never had sex. I thought maybe I really was missing something. (I wasn't.)" [2]

IF YOU'RE A MEMBER OF A CLIQUE OR PEER GROUP, IT IS IMPORTANT TO share likes and dislikes and discourage differences. Young people conform because they don't want to be left out. They want to feel as if they are part of something. They don't want to be laughed at. Nobody wants to be too different from their peers.

Peer groups are also part of becoming independent from your parents. Through your circle of friends, you try on new ideas and behaviors.

But some friends can pressure you to deny your own feelings and thoughts. When you begin to rely on others to tell you what you think, feel, and know, you can become disconnected from your own feelings and values. The more you resist this disconnection from your values, the more you discover yourself and your own strength. Your inner strength is one of the foundations of positive self-respect and a healthy future.

If you disagree with your friends' behavior, you may have to find new friends. This can be difficult, but in the end, you have to live with yourself and the consequences of your actions—for life.

Sexual pressures

Some peer groups place a high premium on virginity. Girls who don't follow this code can get a "bad reputation."

❖

Other groups may view being sexually active as a status symbol. Well-known sex authors Masters and Johnson say, "A new tyranny of sexual values is emerging; teenagers are expected by their peers to become sexually experienced at an early age, and those who are not comfortable with this pressure are viewed as old-fashioned, immature, or 'uptight.' "[3]

❖

Sex is a personal matter. If another teen asks you if you are a virgin, you don't owe them an answer. You don't have to open your private life and feelings to curious spectators who may want to pressure you. Laugh it off with, "Yeah—like I'm going to tell you."

Nobody should pressure you to have sex. Sex is private, and your choice is your business.

❖

In some peer groups, boys encourage their friends to get as much sex as they can as often as possible. But many boys feel anxious and uncomfortable with this pressure to "score" no matter who gets hurt.

Sometimes a boy's own father may push him to get out there and score. A father who puts this kind of burden on his son doesn't realize he may be damaging his son's personality.

When a boy is pressured to go as far sexually as he can, it can end up being a no-win situation. If he doesn't try, he can feel like a failure. If his date lets him, she may feel like a failure.

❖

For some girls, an older boyfriend is a status symbol. But when they come up against the more powerful personalities of boys who are several years older, they may be pushed into situations they're not ready for. Older guys may be more insistent about having sex. Girls should be extremely cautious about dating older guys.

Boys wonder, "What is this going to get me into?"

Boys, too, can feel pressure from girls to have sex. Jeffrey, age sixteen, explains, "You're at a party and you're making out and she wants more. You know what I mean. And you're thinking, 'Wow, what is this going to get me into? I don't want to have a relationship with this chick.' But if you don't go for it, she thinks you're really weird. . . ."[4]

❖

Chance, seventeen, says, "You meet a good-looking girl and you ask her, 'What's happening?' or 'Where do you go to school?' and she's like, 'Are you a virgin?' 'Who are you doing it with?' You can tell what she's looking for, and you start feeling like a piece of meat or something."

❖

Some boys may not feel like having sex. Others know it's wrong to push a girl, or to have sex with a near stranger, or to put their girl-friend at risk of pregnancy or disease. But in their heads they may hear the voices of their friends saying, "What are you? Some kind of wimp? Go for it!" or "Get as much as you can!" or "Act like a man!" or "So what if she said no? She doesn't mean it. Go on!"

A real man

A real man does not have to "score." A real man doesn't feel like he has to prove anything to anybody. He is self-assured about his sexuality. A real man does not push a woman to have sex.

❖

Guys who need to "score" are usually the guys who don't feel very good about themselves and need something to brag about.

❖

A real man gains respect from both sexes by behaving honorably and considerately toward women and by keeping his experiences to himself.

A real woman

If a young woman is strong enough to resist the "everybody's-doing-it-so-why-not?" trend, she stands a good chance of being respected. In one series of interviews conducted with teenage girls for a national magazine, interviewers found that many of those questioned said they respected girls who had the guts not to buckle under to peer pressure. They admired girls who kept their individuality.[5]

❖

A real woman thinks enough of herself to know she doesn't need to push a guy to have sex with her to feel worthwhile. She knows she can stand on her own.

❖

A woman's worth is not based on her sexiness.

❖

"Putting out" is a poor way to try to be popular or raise your self-esteem.

Both sexes need to remember

Sometimes it's hard for girls to remember: What boys think of me has nothing to do with who I really am. I am not on earth to serve a boy, give in to a boy, or live for a boy.

Sometimes it's hard for boys to remember: Whether or not I'm a sexual success with girls at this point in my life is not what's important. Sex can be a real drag on my future.

Keep in mind: You have your whole life ahead of you. You are a person with unique talents. Recognize your abilities. They are yours to develop and to use to make your way in the world. Recognizing your talents is hard work. Do your best in school. Read. Write. Volunteer in your community. Slowly but surely your talents will emerge. Watch for them. Build on them. You'll know what they are because they will be things you like to do and are good at. Don't let sex mess up your future.

Not everyone is doing it

Louisy, sixteen, says, "At one time, I did feel like I was the only virgin on the earth. But then my friend was like, 'Well, you know, I'm a virgin, and she's a virgin and she's a virgin.'

"I could not imagine what it would be like to be a pushover, to be someone who would have sex with your boyfriend just because you would lose him, because that's just the way I am. You cannot pressure me.

"I think that's why I fell in love with Meleke. He's sensitive himself, he's a sensitive guy. He doesn't pressure me at all. His eyes are gorgeous; I could look at his eyes all day."[6]

❖

The truth, of course, is that not everyone is doing it. Even among students at the best-known U.S. colleges and universities, not everyone is doing it. A survey of students age twenty-one and under at the University of California at Los Angeles (UCLA) found that half had never had sexual intercourse.

"I don't think everybody's having sex," says a UCLA political science major named Lee. "I have lots of friends who are virgins."

Tom, a communications student, comments, "I know lots of other people who aren't having sex." He explains, "It's hard being a virgin if you don't want to be, but it's pretty easy to remain one if you want to. No one makes me feel like I have to have sex to be cool or popular. I make the rules for me."

A better way to impress friends

Some girls think that getting pregnant and having a baby is a good way to get special recognition and attention from their friends. But this attention doesn't last long. The more common effect of early motherhood is that the teenage girl will eventually be separated from her friends and isolated from their activities. And she may lose her chance for a better education, which could have made a positive difference in her life. If you find yourself thinking of motherhood as a way to look better in your friends' eyes, consider talking to a school counselor. The counselor can explain how having a baby could affect your social status. They can help you figure out other ways of gaining recognition. Counselors are trained to help you discover what you're good at and how to use your talents and skills so that you'll feel like a valuable part of your school and community.

❖

Likewise, both young men and women need to realize that trying to impress friends by having sex can backfire. Your friends won't be impressed for long, and you may face the life-long consequences of an unplanned pregnancy or disease. It's simply not worth the risk. Why not earn everyone's respect by excelling in academics, a sport, a hobby, volunteer work, or a part-time job?

There are many other ways to impress your friends, and the self-esteem you build will last a lifetime.

"They want me to have sex so they won't feel guilty"

Everybody thinks about sex and many talk about sex, but the truth is that millions of teenagers are virgins.

❖

Sexually active teens often pressure their friends who are virgins. They try to make virgins feel that they've made the wrong decision or aren't cool. As one teenager, Christy, said, "They want me to have sex so they won't feel guilty. I won't help them out that way."[7]

❖

What can you say if a sexually experienced friend pressures you to lose your virginity? You could respond in this way: "I could choose to be like you any day, but you will never be like me again."[8]

❖

If your friends are pushing you to do things that can mess you up, are they the kind of people you should be hanging out with and listening to about important life issues? Friends should help each other make good decisions and look out for each other's futures, not nudge one another into risky and questionable behaviors. Be careful about whose advice you're taking.

Making a phony impression

Some kids who act the most sophisticated about sex are actually the ones who are most worried about it. They love to make a false impression about their attitudes and experience. They love to tell those with less experience that "everybody's doing it." The truth may be that they have lots of anxieties about their decision to have sex, and all the bragging makes them feel better. So when you hear that "everybody's doing it," maybe you're just being fooled by a few kids who aren't telling you the whole truth.

❖

Erika, eighteen, who has decided to remain a virgin until marriage, says a few of her classmates ask her, "How can you still be a virgin?" or "Didn't you ever just feel like letting go with a guy?" or "You must be frustrated." But Erika says, "I'm fine with the way I am. Besides,

I've heard enough stories about what some of these girls have been through. I don't actually think they're having such a good time."

If everybody is doing it . . .

If everybody is doing it, joining in is unwise when you consider that everybody doing it is taking a big chance on getting and spreading sexually transmitted diseases (STDs). The more people have sex with multiple partners, the more diseases are spread. In fact, more than 8,000 teens a day catch an STD.

❖

When you consider that half of teen pregnancies begin during the first six months of sexual activity, you have to ask, "Has everybody who's doing it made a smart choice?"

Make your own choices

It's important to make up your own mind and make your own choices, even if it means bucking the crowd. If young Marie Curie, Abraham Lincoln, Joan of Arc, and Albert Schweitzer had begun by trying to figure out what would be popular with others and doing that, chances are good we'd never have heard their names. [9]

❖

Is not being popular such a curse? While it's no fun watching the so-called "popular" kids from afar and feeling like an outsider, outsiders have some advantages. While the in-crowd is busy being popular, acting popular, maintaining their status, talking themselves up and others down, they may not be doing a lot of growing. Outsiders, on the other hand, can spend their time more thoughtfully and usefully. They can grow emotionally and intellectually. Have you ever heard the saying, "Adversity builds character"? This means that living through hard times makes you a stronger, more interesting human being.

❖

In a recent magazine interview, actor Jaleel White advised young people that the only way to find peace with themselves is to be true to their own values. White added that what everybody thinks is cool today won't seem so cool in a year. [10]

Choose your friends carefully

"I really want to wait," says Morgan, sixteen. "But sometimes I'm afraid I'm the only one who feels that way."

One of the biggest favors you can do for your future self is to have well-adjusted friends now who support your decision to abstain from sex. Stick with the kids who have their heads on straight and their values in the right place.

❖

Best Friends, a highly successful[11] abstinence program for teenage girls in Washington, D.C., helps girls support each other as "best friends." One member commented, "One time I was going to go with this guy who had this great line, but they (the Best Friends girls) wouldn't let me. I'm really glad. He got another friend of mine pregnant and left her alone. She's sad. We watch out for each other."[12]

❖

Christine, another member of Best Friends, says, "Instead of focusing on boys and sex, Best Friends teaches us to get good grades, go to college, and set standards and goals that we want to achieve. . . . People that give in to having sex before they're ready give up their self-control. For me being abstinent is important because I have goals for my life. I want to become a biologist, and there's no way I can do that if I'm having sexual encounters and getting pregnant. I don't want to have sexual relations with anyone until I get married."[13]

❖

If you and your friends share the same views about the benefits of postponing sex, it's likelier you'll wait and that you'll feel more sure your decision is right.

❖

It's important for teens fifteen to eighteen to figure out how they feel about sex and to get their "value system" in order while they're still in high school. If they don't, they may be overwhelmed by the sexual pressures and sexual freedom they encounter on a college campus. Once they get there, they won't have their parents' rules to impose order on their life.

❖

No one expects you to map out your entire future while you're still a teenager. Many young people feel like Serena, who observes, "I change my mind all the time about what I want to be. When I was eleven, I was sure I was going to be an astronaut. Later I decided I wanted to go into politics. A month ago, I told my friends I wanted to have six kids." She adds with a laugh, "Today I can't believe I said that." It's probable that you won't decide just what you want to do in life until you're older. But one of the smartest goals you can have right now is to keep all your options open. This means not doing anything that decreases your future choices. You have read enough in this book to understand that sexual activity can interfere seriously with the plans you're making for your future.

WHAT DO YOU WANT FOR YOUR FUTURE?

Does teen sex fit in with your plans and your life goals? How would you answer the following questions?

- What can I do now and in the future that will make me proud of myself?
- What goals do I have for my life? (A college education or an advanced degree? A career in science, computers, health, education, business? Travel opportunities? Marriage and a family?)
- What values do I believe in? (Are there certain behaviors and ways of living and interacting with others that I think are best?)
- Am I careful about making decisions that will help me live up to my values and goals?

How do the media influence your thinking about sex?

Popular music, advertising, movies, magazines, and TV influence the way teens think about their sexuality. From the media, teens get ideas about what's beautiful or macho, what's sexy or romantic, what's cool, and what's desirable.

❖

In the movies, sex is commonplace. Everybody is jumping into bed with everyone else. Relationships move quickly to intercourse. Sex looks glamorous, intense, and irresistible. After a steady bombardment of these images over the years, it's easy to see sex as the path to romance, excitement, and personal fulfillment.

If you see enough of these images, you might start to think of sex as something that's not only acceptable, but actually expected of you. It's equally hard to ignore the headlines that jump out at you at the check-out counter: "The Secret Sexual You—Turn Her Loose" (*Glamour* cover story) or "What Men Think When They First See You Naked" (*Cosmopolitan* cover story). The media's slick messages about sex can easily drown out messages about waiting that you hear from your parents, teachers, church, or friends. Having sex can appear to be a great way to be popular and to take part in your world.

❖

Are the media really concerned with the quality of your life? No. In fact, their concern lies somewhere quite different. The main purpose of all these sexual images is to make money.

Not only are feature articles and programs full of exciting-looking sex, but often the accompanying advertisements are also sexual. Thus, you are primed to see casual sex as attractive and fulfilling; you are then shown products to enhance your own sexiness. You are made to feel, for example, that only by wearing a certain brand of jeans will you be sexy and valuable, or that you will finally be worth the attention of the opposite sex if you buy a certain exercise machine to lose weight, or build up your muscles, or shape yourself to physical perfection. You are made to feel that your sexiness and desirability can be assured by using a certain brand of cologne.

❖

The media's goal is certainly not to guide you toward healthy relationships or a healthy marriage or help you hold out for the electrifying sexual satisfaction that takes place between adult lifetime partners. The media are not concerned with your long-term happiness, but with molding you to become a consumer of their vision and their products.

When teens buy into the media's vision that having sex and being sexy are necessary for young people to find joy in life, they are being manipulated.

Work on feeling good about yourself

In her book *Reviving Ophelia*, Mary Pipher suggests a number of things teenagers can do to work on feeling strong and good about themselves.[14] The following ideas include some of her suggestions:

- Make a list of all the things about you that are positive and tack it on your bulletin board. Read it each day. At the end of each day, tell yourself all the things you did that day that made you proud.

- Keep a private journal where you write down your thoughts and feelings. Let it be the place where you honestly express your point of view about what happens in your life. Use it to try to make sense of the confusion you may feel.

- Do volunteer work helping people in your community. You'll be amazed at how good you'll feel about yourself. You'll learn more about what you can do, you'll feel like an important part of your community, and you'll stop thinking that you and your problems are alone in the universe.

❖

"Take control of your life," advises a young woman named Sheila. "Make decisions about your life and arrange to make those things happen. If you respect yourself, your decisions and priorities, I find that it generally follows that you don't need another person—you have yourself. And then it seems that it's easier to find and enjoy someone and for that person to enjoy you."[15]

chapter 9

What's the
Double Standard?

Ninth grader Kenny comments, "Where I used to live, the guys had to go out and get laid. . . . There was real pressure on you. . . . If you weren't acting like a sex maniac, everybody thought there was something wrong with you. But it was the opposite for the girls. They heard, 'Stay pure. Save yourself. Don't be cheap.' " [1]

A high school girl explains, "If a girl makes love to a guy one night and it gets around the school, no one looks at him like a sleaze. They think he's macho!" [2]

"The same girls who are pressured to have sex on Saturday night are called sluts on Monday morning. The boys who coaxed them into sex at the parties avoid them in the halls at school," relates psychologist Mary Pipher. [3]

AS CHILDREN GROW, THEIR PARENTS AND OTHERS GRADUALLY MAKE them aware of what they think is proper "role behavior." Role behavior refers to how a boy behaves versus how a girl behaves. For example, parents may buy toy trucks for boys and dolls for girls. They may expect a son to become a doctor and a daughter to become a nurse. Children may see this in their own families: Dad is the powerful one and Mom does what he says. Gradually children gain an impression of how they are to regard their bodies and their interactions with the opposite sex.

In traditional American culture, this role behavior has resulted in the belief that "boys are tough" and "girls are weaker and should give in to boys." In recent decades, we have been trying hard to unlearn this old idea. It is clearly unfair to both women and men. Yet if we are honest and realistic, we have to admit it's a pattern that we're having trouble shaking off. This pattern, as unjust as it is, strongly influences our sexual behavior and sexual outlook. It leads to what is commonly referred to as the "double standard."

According to the double standard, boys have one set of rules about sexuality and girls have another. With this terribly unfair double standard, both sexes may come to believe that sex before marriage is okay for boys but girls who have premarital sex are bad.

She's a slut. He's a stud.

How do we know that the double standard still exists? When you hear negative words like "slut," "sleaze," and "tramp" used to describe girls who have sex, and more positive words like "macho," "stud," "Romeo," or "lover boy" to describe boys, you're hearing the double standard. (Have you ever heard a boy called a slut?)

❖

What's a girl to do? She's caught between the new social pressure to "go for it!" and the old idea that she'll be punished by society if she has sex.

❖

Desperate to be popular or to find love, girls give in to pressures to have sex and then find themselves scorned as "sluts."

❖

Guys have other words they use to describe girls that they think have had sex a lot. They say these girls are "worn out." They also say, "She's been run."[4] This is cruel and unfair, but guys say it.

❖

Often it is girls who trash another girl's reputation. They may label another girl a "slut," " 'ho," "sleaze," or "skank." Instead of defending each other, girls may gossip, criticize, and start rumors. Their victims may become social outcasts.

❖

One girl recalls, "Up until junior year, there were only two girls we knew weren't virgins. We were always going up and asking them these questions [about sex]. Then afterwards we'd talk about them like they were dogs or something."[5]

Girls get "a reputation"

For girls, the double standard can lead to a bad reputation and a lack of self-respect. A bad reputation can wreck a girl's teenage years. Other girls may shun her, and boys may get the wrong idea. If a boy asks her out, she won't know if he likes her for real or because he thinks he'll have an easy time getting her to have sex with him. At first she might like all the attention, but when she figures out that the guys don't really care about her, she'll feel awful. Getting rid of a bad reputation can be hard.

Boys lose self-respect

For boys, the double standard can lead to efforts to score with as many girls as possible and to brag about sexual exploits. It makes boys behave dishonestly toward girls and hurt girls in ways that boys know are wrong. It can make boys lose respect for themselves when they know they've treated other human beings without decency and fairness.

❖

The double standard wrongly tells kids that sex is something girls give and boys take. When a boy and girl are on a date, he is expected to try to go as far as he can and not take "no" for an answer, and she's expected to restrain him. If things go too far, it's her fault. This way of thinking is so unfair that it's hard to believe our culture still buys into it. Yet teens themselves force each other to keep playing the same old game.

"I love you, but I can't see you anymore"

Author Nancy Friday quotes a sixteen-year-old girl who says, "You have to know when to say stop. Otherwise, a guy may suddenly say, 'I love you, but I can't see you anymore.' The girl can't understand why. She's done what he's been begging her to do, but instead of committing himself to her more, suddenly he's backing off."

Friday says what the boy really meant was, "I love you but you have broken one of my secret rules so I'm not going to love you anymore."[6] His "secret rule" is that nice girls don't go around having sex.

Who should behave honorably?

A young man comments, "To have a serious relationship, I have to respect a girl's morals." But shouldn't honorable behavior be the same for both sexes? Boys who believe that holding off on sex is honorable behavior in a girl should see it as honorable behavior in themselves.

❖

Boys who believe in equal rights and equal responsibilities for both sexes can show it by banishing words like "slut," "sleaze," "tramp," and "easy lay" from their vocabulary. They can refuse to brag to their friends about their relationships. They can resolve not to push or coerce girls into having sex. They should be aware of how much the "scoring" mentality hurts girls. And they should stand up for their girlfriends' honor.

❖

Girls, likewise, should stand up for each other, instead of thoughtlessly damaging another's reputation. All of us know how hurtful it is to have someone talk about us behind our backs. And when you really think about it, aren't the girls who are doing the name calling just trying to make themselves feel superior? This says more about *their* character than it does about the girl they're gossiping about.

chapter 10

Sexual Liberation:

Was it really liberating?

The following are comments from young people in the 1960s, the beginning of the era of Sexual Liberation:

A boy explained, "We don't know any more than [girls] do and we're just as scared. Oh, maybe a few of us are into this new sex-freedom business, but believe me, most of us are as frightened of the whole thing as the girls are." [1]

A male college student confided, "I am . . . troubled because I am not really looking for a wife but sort of take advantage of nice girls who assume I am. It is just too much for me to turn down a chance to go all the way." [2]

A young woman commented, "Many men want a girl to say no. They are honestly happy when she does. They want to respect somebody." [3]

"Sometimes I wish I were in college ten years ago when people just dated," said one college woman. "I think I would have been happier." [4]

GROWING UP NOW AND IN THE LAST THIRTY YEARS HAS BEEN UNUSUALLY difficult. Your grandparents lived by strict rules about boy-girl interactions, dating, and sex. Most kids back then didn't question these rules. They thought it was fine to live by the rule, "No sex before marriage." Besides, in those "olden days" lots of young people married in their late teens. (Now the average age of marriage is twenty-five for women and twenty-seven for men.) This made their lives simpler than yours. They didn't have to face the worries that go along with premarital sex and multiple partners.

But in the 1960s something called "Sexual Liberation," or the "Sexual Revolution," hit. This began a period when rules about sexual behavior were relaxed and young men and women on college campuses began to experiment with sex. It was a time of pressure to act sexually liberated. Liberation means freedom, but many remember it as a time of heartbreak and unhappiness.

A lot of pain

One woman recalls, "Most of my friends came to college as virgins, and all of us lost our virginity there, usually in our second year. But most of us ended up in very troubled, rocky, unsatisfactory relationships. There was a lot of pain. There [was] . . . a lot of trying something out for one night and then feeling awful about it the next morning. There was none of the rollicking fun, joviality, and freeness and nudity that was supposed to be going on. There was just a lot of sh—."[5]

❖

Another says, "I felt pressured to prove I was a liberated woman and could do whatever I wanted—even though most of the time I really didn't want to be sleeping with the men I was proving myself to. I didn't learn to say no until I was thirty—that was truly liberating."[6]

❖

Although the sexual revolution began on college campuses, it's now found in high schools and junior highs. Kids today are facing decisions about sex at an earlier age. Many don't realize that messing with sex is messing with your head. Teens may say, "We're old enough to handle sex." But after a while, some realize how much pressure they're under and are sad about giving up their happy times of just being a kid.

❖

If you feel pressured by your friends to participate in sexual liberation, are you really free? Or are you actually giving up the freedom to make choices that might be better for you?

A disaster for girls

"The new sexual revolution has been a disaster for girls," writes one researcher. Girls bear the heavy burdens of the revolution—pregnancy, sexual abuse and coercion from older boys or men, abortion, teen motherhood, poverty, and diseases that can lead to infertility.

Because of the sexual revolution, it's a lot harder for girls to say no. Female goals of intimacy and commitment have given way to the old male goal of sex with no strings attached.[7]

"I hope I never get that serious!"

When you compare your life with your parents' lives, don't you sometimes think, "I hope I never get that serious!"?

If you become sexually active, things get serious fast. Your fun gets more and more adult until it's no fun anymore. Before long, you feel like the weight of the world is on your shoulders, like your youth is over—way too soon.

Do you win or lose?

You can be "sexually liberated" and still be tongue-tied with your date. You can be "sexually liberated" and not know what a good sexual experience involves. You can be "sexually liberated" and still be confused about when to have sex. You can be "sexually liberated" and still not know how and why to say no. You can be "sexually liberated" and still wonder how you could have been so stupid. And you can be "sexually liberated" and find yourself the prisoner of a broken heart.

❖

A law student named Bob makes the comment, "So many kids in my generation got fooled into thinking they were liberated, but the fact is they lost out on the excitement that comes with saving sex for marriage."

Fifteen years of love affairs

The following letter to Ann Landers shows how one woman's life was deeply affected by the sexual revolution.

103

Dear Ann:

I am a forty-three-year-old mother of a teenage daughter. I have been divorced since she was two. I never meant to be promiscuous, but fifteen years of love affairs can make a record look pretty bad. Each new affair was meant to be the 'affair to end all affairs.' Each new lover was expected to be the key to my happiness and the solution to all my problems. Because of this attitude (which I have since changed) I became involved in sexual relationships too eagerly and too soon. Then I would end up getting hurt or hurting the man.

I realize now that men are always ready and eager to have sex. I don't believe most of them intentionally hurt or exploit women, but if a woman is too willing and too eager to please, a man finds it difficult to understand that she could want more from him than just a good time in bed.

It's taken a long time, but I'm finally willing to admit that our mothers and grandmothers weren't just prudes, they were SMART. In their day, couples went through a courtship or dating period that enabled them to get to know each other before becoming sexually involved. I'm sure this saved a lot of pain and grief and made for stable and lasting relationships. Today, the sexual revolution notwithstanding, it's still up to the woman to have enough self-respect and self-control to set limits and decide for herself if and when she wants to say "yes." My daughter already knows this. Thank goodness her mother does, too.

—Happier and Wiser [8]

chapter 11

Your Personal Policy on Sex

"It just happened."

"It was our emotions."

"We couldn't help ourselves."

"We were swept away."

THE VIEW THAT ROMANTIC LOVE IS SOMETHING IRRESISTIBLE, SOMETHING that magically makes us lose our heads and behave uncontrollably, is a dangerous trap. It excuses us from making decisions about our actions and passions.

The decisions you make about sex set the stage for your entire life. If you make good decisions, you safeguard your future. You are likely to establish a strong identity that will serve you well for a lifetime. But if you blow it, if you let sex "just happen," if you flip-flop from one sexual relationship to another, you weaken yourself and your ability to take a forceful position on future choices about sex and other areas of your life. For example, if you are strong and secure in your values and goals, you will be more likely to stand up to peer pressure, complete your education, and remain honest and ethical in your career.

Stumbling into sex

About 75 percent of boys and 83 percent of girls say they did not plan their "first time."[1] By stumbling into their first sexual encounter, they risked pregnancy, disease, and emotional hurt. And they wasted their first time.

❖

Author Nancy Friday refers to the "almost suicidally foolish manner in which [young] women enter sex"[2] without protection. Of course, it is "suicidally foolish" for young men as well.

Most of these teens thought they'd make up their minds about sex as they went along. No wonder the rates of teen pregnancy and disease are so high. Many young people just don't use their heads.

❖

Your intelligence and powers of reasoning need to play a big role in making decisions about sex. When you throw away your opportunity to decide about sex, you lose the ability to take charge of your life.

Your Personal Policy on sexual activity

Making decisions about how you will handle your sexuality takes a long time. It may take many days, weeks, or months of thinking about yourself, your values, and your goals and weighing all this against how you believe sexual activity could affect you.

It's not something you can do on the spur of the moment, in the middle of a passionate love affair. It's something you need to have firmly in mind way ahead of time. Right now, start thinking about a policy that's right for you.

❖

Use this book to help you understand many of these complicated issues. You will eventually come up with your own Personal Policy about sex. Because it will be YOUR policy based on your reasoning, you will be much more likely to stick with it.

How do I come up with my Personal Policy?

Arriving at a Personal Policy means that you will define *personal goals* for your life, devise *personal rules* to help you stay on track, and outline a *personal course of action* that will help you reach your goals.

Here is an example of the kind of thinking that will help you start making reasonable decisions about sex. Since sex often results in unplanned pregnancy, you might examine your views about children's needs. For example, do you believe that children deserve a stable family with mature, loving parents? If so, then this belief can guide you in making decisions. If you keep in mind that no method of birth control is 100 percent effective, and that teens often don't use birth control even though they know better, you'll understand there is a very real chance of accidental pregnancy for teenagers. If you read chapters 5 and 7, you learned how teen sex can hurt the life of an innocent child. A Personal Policy of postponing sex until you're much older places a value on children's lives.

Ask yourself these questions

Here are some other questions to think about. They will help you decide whether teen sex has a place in your life and your goals.

- How would I feel about having to choose between abortion, adoption, or raising a child?
- Am I ready to give up my freedom to parent a child?
- Can I afford to raise and support a child?
- What if I had to pay hundreds of dollars every month in child support until I am middle-aged?
- If my partner and I were faced with an unplanned pregnancy, how would our relationship be affected? How would our families be affected?
- How would my education and chance at a good career be affected by a pregnancy?
- If I got a sexually transmitted disease, what would happen to my health? How would I feel about myself?
- If I began having sex with my partner, and they walked out on the relationship, how would I be affected? What if this happened several times—as it does to most sexually active teens?
- Is there something special about my virginity?
- Deep in my heart and mind, do I think teen sex is right or wrong, moral or immoral?
- Do I "live for the moment" without thinking of how my behavior might hurt me later on, or do I carefully consider the consequences of my actions?
- Do I believe that sex should take place only with a serious, long-term commitment from both partners?

- Do I assume that a sexual relationship will create a long-term commitment?
- How can I live my life now in order to give myself the best possible chance for a successful future?

Try writing brief responses to these questions. Then write a one-page summary of your feelings about teen sex, including whether you think postponing sex until you are older is a good idea.

❖

The following is an example of a Personal Policy—goals, rules, and course of action—based on responses to the questions on the previous page. Your own policy will reflect your own personal views.

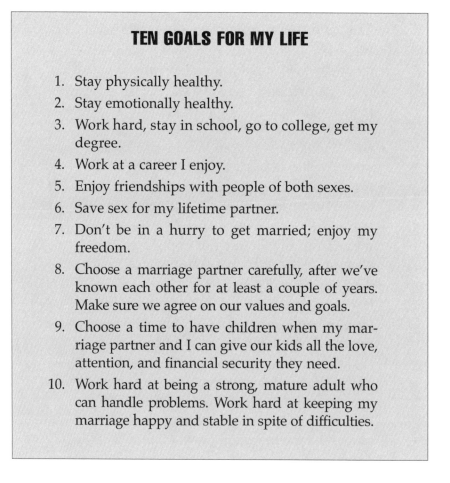

TEN GOALS FOR MY LIFE

1. Stay physically healthy.
2. Stay emotionally healthy.
3. Work hard, stay in school, go to college, get my degree.
4. Work at a career I enjoy.
5. Enjoy friendships with people of both sexes.
6. Save sex for my lifetime partner.
7. Don't be in a hurry to get married; enjoy my freedom.
8. Choose a marriage partner carefully, after we've known each other for at least a couple of years. Make sure we agree on our values and goals.
9. Choose a time to have children when my marriage partner and I can give our kids all the love, attention, and financial security they need.
10. Work hard at being a strong, mature adult who can handle problems. Work hard at keeping my marriage happy and stable in spite of difficulties.

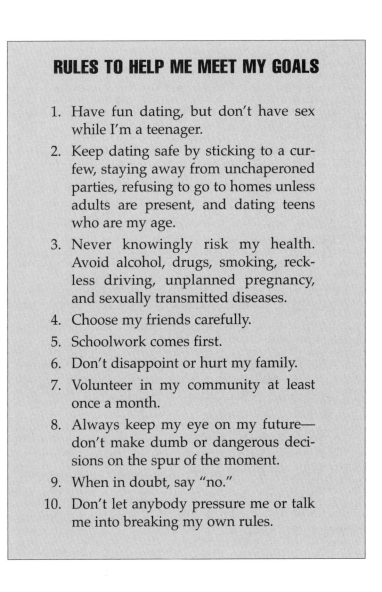

RULES TO HELP ME MEET MY GOALS

1. Have fun dating, but don't have sex while I'm a teenager.
2. Keep dating safe by sticking to a curfew, staying away from unchaperoned parties, refusing to go to homes unless adults are present, and dating teens who are my age.
3. Never knowingly risk my health. Avoid alcohol, drugs, smoking, reckless driving, unplanned pregnancy, and sexually transmitted diseases.
4. Choose my friends carefully.
5. Schoolwork comes first.
6. Don't disappoint or hurt my family.
7. Volunteer in my community at least once a month.
8. Always keep my eye on my future— don't make dumb or dangerous decisions on the spur of the moment.
9. When in doubt, say "no."
10. Don't let anybody pressure me or talk me into breaking my own rules.

MY PERSONAL COURSE OF ACTION
TO HELP ME REACH MY GOALS

1. I will try to date only partners who accept or support my views about postponing sex.
2. I will work out a curfew and other dating guidelines with my parents.
3. I will stay active, eat healthy, get lots of exercise, sleep enough, and find hobbies I enjoy that keep me busy in my spare time.
4. I will seek best friends who will support my views on holding off on sex and living a healthy life.
5. I will set aside time everyday for homework. I will work hard at making good grades.
6. I will help my parents, try to respect their point of view, and ask their advice when something comes up that I can't handle.
7. I will ask a teacher, a social agency, or a priest, rabbi, or other religious leader about the kinds of volunteer jobs available that will help me become a valuable part of my community.
8. When I suspect that an activity is unwise, I will think hard about my hopes for the future, and I will carefully consider the possible consequences.
9. I will talk with my friends, parents, or counselor to figure out the best ways to say "no."
10. I will practice being the kind of person who cannot be pushed around, dared, or pressured into doing something I think is bad for me. I will practice standing up for my point of view and explaining my ideas.

Now that you have read someone else's Personal Policy, try writing down your own goals, rules, and plan of action. Write down as many items under each category as you are comfortable with. Read your lists from time to time and revise your Personal Policy if necessary.

Your Personal Power

By setting your own goals, making your own rules, and sticking to them, you are exercising your Personal Power—your ability to take charge of your own life. With this power comes self-respect and self-confidence. The more you behave according to your beliefs, values, and goals, the better chance you have of being self-confident and successful. You will demonstrate to yourself and others that you have power over what happens in your life.

The reverse is also true. The more you abandon your beliefs and values and engage in activities you don't feel right about, the less you'll respect yourself. Not only will your actions cause you guilt and regret, but you'll also be less confident about your judgment. You may come to believe that what happens to you in life is out of your control, a feeling that leads to failure.

❖

Once you have figured out your Personal Policy on sex, you will have a framework for living up to your values and goals.

❖

Are you going to follow your internal compass? Are you going to decide on your own Personal Policy? Are you going to exercise your Personal Power to take control of your life? Or are you going to stumble through life, letting things "just happen" to you?

....

chapter 12

Why Choose Abstinence?

A young man who is committed to postponing sex until marriage asks, "What could be more exciting, more special, more emotional than sharing the wonders of sex with your one true and dedicated love?" [1]

A sexually active sixteen-year-old says, "My fantasy has always been to wait . . . until my honeymoon and have it on one of those huge beds with nice sheets. Or in one of those baths with lots of bubbles. I think it's great to do it for the first time with your husband. My fantasy is to have waited." [2]

"If we do get married," says David of his petite, blond girl-friend, "the thing I would cherish most—besides the fact that I was married to her—is that on our first night, I could look her square in the eye and say, 'This was so important to me that I give this to you. You are the first and only one I will ever sleep with.' That, I think, is an incredible gift." [3]

ABSTINENCE MEANS NOT HAVING SEXUAL INTERCOURSE AT ALL. NO genital-to-genital contact. It means no oral or anal sex. It does not mean no hugging, kissing, or cuddling.

Virginity is absolutely normal, not old-fashioned. And it certainly doesn't mean a girl is frigid (not interested in sex) or a boy isn't masculine.

"I look at virginity as a gift to be honorably saved for that one person you decide to spend your lifetime with," says one boy on an Internet forum. "[It's] the greatest emotional and physical treasure a person can give. You don't take it. You don't lose it. You give it. Isn't that what true love is about?" [4]

To do it or not to do it

The decision to become sexually active as a teen is like agreeing to ride an emotional roller coaster. On the upside, there can be a period of emotional highs and physical pleasure. On the downside, there's anxiety about your sexual performance and the appearance of your body, worries about rejection, eventual rejection, anguish, depression, feelings of confusion and worthlessness, and an inability to concentrate on anything but your troubles. There's also intense fear of pregnancy, disease, and AIDS.

❖

"A lot of my friends . . . have gotten pregnant or gotten an STD, and they tell me about the situation," says Sharon, sixteen. "They say things like 'I was so into him I just couldn't stop.' I was like, 'Look, you have to stop; just one time could change your whole life.' "[5]

❖

Some teens (and some adults) think that high moral standards and virtuous behavior are old-fashioned or just plain dumb. They think that these values are suitable only for people who are immature, weak, geeky, uncool, or uninspired. They think of themselves as special, out-of-the-ordinary beings who should take advantage of other, freer, "lifestyle" choices.

According to radio talk show host and columnist Dr. Laura Schlessinger, "Every day on my radio program, I talk with people who have gotten themselves into all sorts of troubled, unhappy and unworkable situations because they put aside what was sensible, good, right, legal, moral or holy and turned instead to what they thought were worthy, viable alternatives."[6] Trying out alternative values or morals can lead to calamity and pain.

❖

A decision to abstain from sexual intercourse leaves you free to make a success of your life, live up to your goals and values, and prepare for a stable, loving, mature partner who will be true to you.

❖

A decision to abstain gives you the freedom to learn to communicate better with friends of the opposite sex.

❖

You have a lot of growing up to do before you get married. During your teenage years, you're getting ready for the right time with the right person.[7]

❖

Some teens say to themselves, "Okay, I'll practice abstinence. That is, until someone special comes along." This is missing the point.

The idea is to make a commitment to yourself that you will live your life consistent with your goals, values, and hopes for the future—as if your whole life depended on it.

❖

A teen named Kati addresses other young women on the Internet: "Many of us will fall in love for the first time in high school with some guy. And when we do we'll think that he is the ONE and that we're going to get married and will have three children—Peter, Nicholas, and Cassidy. We'll live in a big blue house with a white picket fence in Beverly Hills.

"So because you love this man so much," she continues, "you have made the ultimate decision to have sex with him. For you, this is the almighty thing that you could do to show your love and affection for him. But what he's thinking is, 'Yah, man, I get to have sex!'

"Okay, now don't get me wrong. I'm not saying that every guy feels this way, but you have to admit, a lot do. For lots of guys, sex is just this thing they do for a good time, not necessarily to show love and affection. That is the reason prostitution has been around for so long.

"After having sex thrown into a relationship, there are so many risks that a majority of teens don't fully understand." She asks, "If you're so positive that you'll be together forever, why not wait to have sex? When you guys get married, you'll still have ninety years to have sex.

"I'm only warning you that only 1 percent of high school sweethearts get married, and 50 percent of those get divorced (I got that off *Oprah*), so your chances are slim."

Kati adds, "For now, just wait and see what happens because most likely you'll end up breaking up and totally not liking him within a year. So why waste such a wonderful thing on someone that in six or seven months you may detest?"[8]

Looking for a relationship that will last

If you're a guy and a virgin, there are hundreds of thousands like you.

❖

In a letter to advice columnist "Dear Abby," a twenty-seven-year-old male virgin wrote in support of a previous letter writer, a young woman who was being pressured for sex by men who wanted a "test drive" before making a bigger commitment to her. She was determined to save sex for marriage. In his letter, the man commented that a marriage had better be built on a more solid foundation than sex, because the sex will eventually, naturally slow down. If the marriage is based on sex, he wrote, a couple might as well plan for a divorce at the same time they plan their wedding. When two virgins marry, sex will only deepen their relationship, he observed.[9]

Who needs the worry?

Guys who get caught up in sex too early may miss a lot in life. Who needs the worry and pressure? Right now, concentrate on all the positive things in your life—friends, studies, sports, family activities, and special interests. You have an entire lifetime ahead of you during which you can enjoy sex.

"Just to be with her"

Sixteen-year-old Greg explains, "The big goal for me is just to be with the girl I like, not to do anything in particular or get any place, just to be with her."[10]

❖

There are hundreds of other romantic, sensual ways to express affection that don't involve sex: cuddling, taking walks in the moonlight, flirting, giving each other small gifts, planning an outing you'll both enjoy, writing love notes, and sharing your deepest thoughts. (For more suggestions, see chapter 13.)

You can both enjoy your time together a lot more when the pressure to have sex is off.

What do you tell your girlfriend?

What if your girlfriend is hinting that she wants to go all the way? Chances are good that she'll respect you a lot if you can explain to her a few of the reasons why you're against it. For example:

- You're not ready to be a father and she's not ready to be a mother.
- Since no means of birth control is 100 percent effective, the only way to be sure you won't bring an unplanned baby into the world is not to have sex.
- Where's the romance in worrying yourselves sick that she might be pregnant?
- The best way to really get to know each other is to leave sex out of it.
- Sex can mess up your relationship. (See chapter 2.)
- You like her too much to do anything that would risk her happiness.

❖

It's possible for a young man and woman to be totally in love and NOT go all the way. It happens all the time! According to these young couples, they've developed a deeper attachment than couples who are sexually involved.

The ultimate act of love

A newspaper article describes the determination of a young couple who have decided to remain virgins until marriage:

Anne and David have "been going together more than four months, and they still haven't taken the magic tumble. They're not going to. Not now, not next week, not if they get sloppy drunk, not even if they get engaged. When the vows are sworn, when the limo driver has whisked them away from the reception, when David has carried Anne across the threshold of the honeymoon suite and laid her gently down on the conjugal bed; then, and only then, it can happen." [11] (David is quoted at the beginning of this chapter.)

❖

Michael, who recently married as a virgin, explains, "When you give yourself to someone in sex, that's the ultimate act, you can't become any closer biologically or emotionally. It's one of the most intimate, maybe *the* most intimate act you can perform. So if you wait until marriage, you're committing to the person that you do marry, that you've never given this part of yourself to anybody before. That is the ultimate act of love.

"It's not hard to abstain from sex or to do anything that you want to do when you have the power in your own psyche . . . to make those decisions. Part of it is self-control and self-discipline. But a better way to describe it would be just a commitment to yourself." [12]

Can teen sex affect your later marriage?

Partners who have had premarital sex are less likely to have happy marriages, contends sociologist Ray Short. [13] Short quotes studies that show that such marriages are more likely to end in divorce for a number of reasons.

❖

Partners who had premarital sex are more than twice as likely to commit adultery (have sex with someone outside of their marriage) after they are married. As a result, their marriages are undermined by suspicions, lack of harmony, and by one partner's discovery of the other's lack of faithfulness. [14]

❖

One effect of premarital sex is that later on, sex within marriage may seen less exciting. Partners may have relished the premarital thrill of getting away with something forbidden so much that they come to miss this excitement. Married sex may seem dull by comparison. This letdown may push partners to try to relive this thrill through adultery, Short explains. This puts their marriage at great risk. [15]

❖

Couples who had sex before marriage are less likely to be satisfied with their married sex lives. One partner may compare the other's sexual abilities or responses with those of previous partners. Even though their marriage partner has normal responses and normal sexual skills, they may think longingly of the wildly erotic behavior of some previous lover and feel cheated and unhappy. [16]

❖

Dating couples who can't hold off on sex may be blinded by it, writes Short. The intensity of the sex can fool them into thinking they're meant for each other. Only after they are married do they discover that the main thing holding them together was sex.[17]

❖

Premarital sex can cause one or the other marriage partner to be sexually "inhibited"—unable to share and enjoy sex freely and fully. This may be because when they had premarital sex, one partner felt guilty about doing something wrong. (See "Guilt and teens" on page 44.) Every time that partner had premarital sex, it was associated with guilt and shame. Even after marriage, the partner continues to think of sex as something bad. Such a marriage partner just can't "let go" and enjoy sex as freely as they could have if sex had been postponed until marriage. It may take years to get over this bad feeling. Sex counselors say this is an extremely common problem and leads to less happy marriages.[18]

❖

Sociologist Short believes that another reason premarital sex breaks up marriages is that it robs couples of the "sexual cement" that can hold them together. He explains that the first years of a marriage are the roughest period of adjustment for a young couple. This is when a marriage is most likely to break up. He says that the first year or two that a couple begins having sex is the most thrilling sexually. If this period of exciting sex occurs during the same year or so that they are going through the difficult early period of adjusting to marriage and each other, then good sex can cement their love and marriage. However, if they had a year or so of premarital sex, then "that precious bonding of sex that could have helped hold them together while they worked out their problems has been largely lost."[19]

❖

Couples may be pushed into a bad marriage by guilt over sex. If two people think they are in love, and if they become engaged, they may decide that sex is finally okay, but only because they are doing it with the one they will marry. However, if either partner later feels there are good reasons for breaking off the engagement, they may feel obligated to go ahead and marry because they have shared the gift of their virginity.

(One out of every three engaged couples breaks off the engagement before marrying, Short explains.)[20]

❖

"My mom and dad waited until they were married, and seeing how much they love each other now after all those years makes me want that for my marriage," says one eighteen-year-old.

❖

A young women named Kristen says that if both partners are virgins on their wedding night, "there will be an incredible feeling of trust and closeness like no other."

She adds, "I am so sick of hearing all that crap about 'you need to know [your partner] in every aspect before you get married.' Well, if you want to know how your mate will be in bed, you can measure them by the level of passion in their kisses and in the way they treat you."[21]

❖

When it comes to sexual compatibility, almost any couple who love each other can achieve a happy sex life, writes Short. He states that the best sex is married sex.

Having premarital sex to test your compatibility can spoil things. You're not shopping for a sex object. You're looking for a lifetime partner and best friend.[22]

Secondary virginity

Sex is not necessarily a wonderful experience when you're young. Feeling awful after a failed sexual relationship has convinced many teens that their decision to have sex was a mistake. Many choose to postpone further sexual activity until they're older. While they can never recapture their virginity, they are said to be choosing "secondary virginity." For many, there is great relief in this decision.

Once you've made your decision, avoid risky situations

Once you've made a decision to abstain from sex, be careful not to let yourself be put in a tempting situation. Remember that heavy making out or petting, heavy drinking or drug use, and lots of unsupervised time alone in either partner's home can lead unexpectedly to sexual intercourse. If you're serious about sticking to your decision to abstain, give yourself a mental pep talk and then walk away from situations you know will tempt you.

❖

Teens shouldn't tease their dates and make them sexually excited when they have no intention of having sex. It's certainly okay to be affectionate, but if your date misunderstands your affection, you should let them know, "I like you, but I want you to understand that I don't want things to go any further." If they don't get it, you should repeat exactly the same words—like a broken record. If you have to say this more than several times, your date is not someone you should trust at all.

❖

Both boys and girls need to be prepared to fend off aggressive dates who want sex and don't want to take no for an answer. For responses that can cool things down, see pages 142 through 143.

❖

Studies show that most first sexual encounters take place in the boy's or girl's home or a friend's home. If you are resolved not to have sex, don't be in someone's home unless a parent is supervising.

❖

Hang out with friends who share your decision to abstain from sex. Instead of pressure, you'll feel support for your decision.

❖

If your parents haven't set a curfew for you, set one for yourself.[23] Being able to say truthfully that you have a curfew may get you out of some awkward situations.

If you're shy, you're at risk

Do you always do what your friends or boyfriend or girlfriend wants to do? Teens who are shy about expressing their wants and standing up for their point of view are at risk of giving in too easily to their partner's sexual pressure. They are also at greater risk of being talked into unprotected sex, which leads to pregnancy and diseases like gonorrhea, syphilis, or AIDS.

❖

If you are the shy type, abstinence can be an important cornerstone of your teen years. A well-considered, rock-solid decision to abstain from sex can protect you when you find yourself being pressured by someone with a stronger personality.

Looking for a marriage partner

Many adults in their twenties who are ready to settle down and marry do not want a partner who has had lots of sex. It goes beyond the secret longing of some to marry a virgin. In this era of AIDS and STDs, the more sexual partners you've had, the less desirable you are to a potential husband or wife.

One man who waited

There are many reasons why postponing sex until you're married is a wise idea. In her book for teenagers, author Lynda Madaras quotes one man, Charlie, who explains his reasons particularly well:

"My wife and I waited until we were married to have sex. . . . I think it was a good decision. Maybe if we'd had sex with other people or with each other before we were married, we'd have been more experienced or knowledgeable. But learning about sex together made it that much more special. We didn't have to worry if either of us was as good as the other lovers either of us might have had before.

"By being willing to wait until we were married, I felt I was showing my wife that it wasn't just sex that I wanted from her but real, true love and a lifelong commitment. And she was showing me the same thing. We really trusted each other, and that made us feel safe enough to really let go. We didn't have to worry that if we did it wrong or it wasn't great the first time that it would be all over. And, in fact, it wasn't so great the first time. It was kind of awkward and embarrassing. But I knew and she knew that we'd both be around tomorrow. This trust and commitment made us able to grow to be better lovers than we might otherwise have been." [24]

....

chapter 13

There Are Many Other Ways to "Make Love"

Myong, twenty, recalls, "I had a steady boyfriend when I was seventeen. We loved each other and got along great. We even talked about getting married. We were physically close, too. My boyfriend wanted to have sex, but he was a sweet guy and he understood when I told him I wasn't ready. He was disappointed, but it didn't ruin the relationship. We had some great times together. I'm glad I waited because we eventually split up. This year, I met someone new that I really care about. I remember my first romance as something very special, and I hope my old boyfriend does too."

Another teen comments, "Sex is overrated. My boyfriend and I have both had sex in other relationships, which all ended badly, and we've been going out for almost eight months, and we still haven't had sex. If we do get married, there will be that experience for us to share. There are other ways to be close in a relationship. . . ." [1]

"My boyfriend and I talked about sex because I wanted him to understand that I want to wait," says a high school senior. "He actually said that he loves me too much to have sex with me."

A seventeen-year-old from New York says, "I could O.D. on affection. I could go with a guy just for affection, no sex, for just kissing and being close. I could do that forever. And affection can be sexy." [2]

Another adds, "I'd be more satisfied with that than any kind of sex." [3]

MANY TEENAGERS TURN TO SEXUAL INTERCOURSE BECAUSE THEY WANT to get physically close to someone—to be cuddled, to feel warmth and affection.

What many young people may not have figured out is that there are *so many ways* to be physically and emotionally close that are more sensual and romantic than intercourse.

You should not be expected to ignore your sexual feelings. They are definitely there, and expressing these feelings adds excitement and joy to your life. But you can be a sexual being without having sexual intercourse. As you explore your sexuality, keep in mind that you have hundreds of "sexual options" that don't involve intercourse. If you have a nagging doubt about being ready for sex, listen hard to that inner voice. Keep in mind that falling in love and feeling sexually attracted are the most thrilling feelings of all.

Other ways to please your lover

Many sexual experiences can be enjoyed without losing your virginity. These experiences are more pleasurable when both partners understand that they are not intended to stimulate feelings that would lead to intercourse.

❖

If a guy feels rejected because his partner doesn't want to have sex with him, he needs to understand that her affection and her acceptance of him can be expressed in many ways.

❖

If you and your partner are in love, and you think that sexual intercourse would be a poor idea, here are a few of the hundreds of ways you can share your sexual attraction and affection: hug, snuggle, kiss, caress, hold hands, walk in the moonlight, watch a beautiful sunset, have a candlelight dinner, run in the rain, say I love you, look at each other's baby pictures, buy your partner a small but thoughtful gift, wear something nice that you know your partner likes, and volunteer together on a meaningful project in your community.

More ways to please your lover

Consider these other suggestions for having fun, expressing affection, and strengthening your relationship:

- If your city has bike paths, choose a route together and spend the afternoon biking.
- Care for each other if you get sick.
- Choose a delicious recipe and cook it together.
- Share a secret about your personality that lets your partner understand you better.
- Jog or work out together.
- Plan a picnic. Shop together, create the meal, choose a favorite place, then enjoy yourselves.
- Schedule a day of sightseeing.
- Check out a book from the library and take turns reading to each other.
- Baby-sit together. Be 100 percent responsible.
- Give each other a silly, private nickname.
- Read your horoscopes together and discuss whether or not they make sense.
- Plan a hike in the woods.
- Send each other a package of goodies.
- Share favorite childhood memories.
- Play footsie.
- Make a pizza together.
- Fly a kite.
- Learn to play "Chopsticks" on the piano. Make beautiful music together.
- Dance cheek to cheek.
- Laze away the afternoon sipping iced tea or soda, arm in arm on an old-fashioned porch swing, sharing your thoughts.
- Help each other with homework.

- Have a summer business together. What about dog walking, plant tending or watering for vacationers, grass mowing, car washing, or baby-sitting?
- Play mind-reading games.
- Send your loved one a perfumed love letter.
- Dedicate a song to your partner on the radio.
- Take turns sending each other letters that describe a quality you admire most in the other.
- Hide a love note in your partner's math book.
- Share your greatest worries—and your biggest dreams.
- Choose, construct, and paint a model car together.
- Make an abstract water-color painting together.
- Write a poem or a song together.
- Ask an elderly neighbor if there's an errand or some yard work that the two of you can do to help out.
- If your town has a Habitat for Humanity group, see if you both can join other volunteers building a house for a needy family.
- On your partner's birthday, send their mom a thank-you note.
- Plan a video night. Each partner can share an old favorite that touched their heart.
- Wash the car together.
- Buy a disposable, preloaded camera, go to a beautiful place, and take pictures of each other having fun.
- Visit a museum of art or natural history.
- Write and send a letter to the President about a national issue that the two of you feel strongly about. Write from the heart. Who knows? Maybe he'll quote you in an upcoming speech. It's happened.
- Together, write a letter to the editor of your city newspaper about a local issue you care about. Chances are excellent that it will be published.

- Plan a barbecue and invite both your families.
- Tell each other your most embarrassing moment.
- Give your partner a compliment at least once a day.
- Learn something new together. Go to the library and choose a topic (for example, computers, animals, music, business, astronomy, movie making, or how to build a house). Become experts on your topic.
- Sit on a hilltop and look for shapes in the clouds.
- If you go out of town, send a postcard every day you're away.
- Learn how to design your own Internet page in cyberspace. Tell the world whatever you want. You might, for example, call your site "Jacob's and Haley's View of Life and Reality." Ask a teacher or librarian for help getting started.
- Write "I Love You" in the dust on your partner's car.
- Build a tree house in the summer.
- Tell your partner what it was about him or her that attracted you in the first place.
- Give a homemade birthday card you created.
- Do each other favors.
- Share a banana split or an ice cream soda.
- Gaze deeply into each other's eyes.
- Start a Memory Box of your time together. In it you might put movie ticket stubs, photos, pebbles from your picnic spot, small locks of hair, pressed flowers, your fingerprints, the words to a favorite song or poem, and other mementos.
- Treat the one you love with respect.
- Whisper sweet nothings.
- Hold each other tight.
- Say you care.

All these things are ways of "making love" and growing close.

A bond of affection

"Romantic rituals of their own devising" fill the days and nights of seventeen-year-olds Tony and Tara who live in a small city in California. The two have been going together for four years. Their relationship does not include sexual intercourse. Tara says proudly, "Tony's not like the other guys I know, who always want to have sex." The two say they feel a bond of affection and understanding that is greater than that felt by couples having intercourse.[4]

❖

When a relationship involves intercourse, there may be so much emphasis on sex and the problems it causes that there isn't enough time for activities like those just mentioned. Teen couples who get caught up in sex too young may never be as close as those who express their affection in these other ways.

❖

Another wonderful thing about the many other ways to "make love" is that neither partner has to worry about pregnancy or AIDS.

Relieving sexual tension

Some of the ideas mentioned on pages 124 through 127 can relieve sexual tension, which, for young people, can be pretty over-whelming. Sexual tension refers to strong sexual feelings and urges that can lead to frustration and physical discomfort. These feelings are what lead some young people into sexual intercourse before they're really ready. A normal way that many people relieve sexual tension is called masturbation: sexual self-stimulation. By the age of twenty-one, about 90 percent of men and women have explored their sexuality in this harmless and natural way.[5] It caus-es no diseases and nobody has gotten pregnant masturbating.

❖

Although most people and churches today have come to accept this private activity, some parents are still giving their kids con-fusing messages about it. This is because their parents confused them. In past generations, parents told their children that mastur-bation could cause acne, insanity, feeble-mindedness, dark circles under the eyes, hair on the palms of one's hands, stunted growth, frigidity, perversions, weakness, blindness, or death. Whew! None of this is true, and it sure didn't stop young people from doing it. It just made them feel scared and guilty. So if you've gotten the idea from your parents that there's something wrong with masturbation, it may just be that they're a little confused about what to say about it and what to think about it.

❖

Self-stimulation can relieve sexual tension, give teens mastery over their sexual impulses, show what sensations bring pleasure and what sensations bring about orgasm (otherwise some girls wouldn't know), and help boys understand how to postpone orgasm during sex. Author Alex Comfort calls masturbation "the natural way of testing the equipment."[6]

❖

A negative aspect of masturbation is that certain people who do it are going to feel guilty about it, no matter what. For them, it may be a poor choice. If you seriously feel that it's a sin, or if you worry a lot about it, it's likely to make you feel bad about yourself. This can be damaging to your mental health.

❖

Another possible negative aspect of masturbation is that too much of it may isolate you. A good thing about our sexual urges is the way they push us out into the world to learn to develop relationships with the opposite sex.

❖

The busier you are with sports, friendships, academics, church activities, or hobbies, the less you'll suffer from sexual tension.

A few words about heavy petting

One substitute for intercourse that isn't a good idea is "heavy petting" (touching each other's genitals) because it so often leads to actual intercourse.

❖

When a couple gets involved in heavy petting, neither may be quite sure how far things will go. One may want the petting to proceed to intercourse and the other may not. (This could lead to date rape.) Or both may get carried away and end up having unprotected sex, which they may regret.

❖

According to sex educator Akagi, during heavy petting the "body's natural, physiological response is to have intercourse. . . . It's often difficult to stop yourself from going all the way—regardless of how moral or religious you are or how frightened you may be of AIDS, pregnancy, or STDs."[7]

Put on the brakes

Eighteen-year-old Jan points out that it's important to learn to put on the brakes when making out. While you may worry that you're "ruining the moment," she says, "You have to learn how to say no before things go too far, or you may end up doing something you're sorry about."

❖

Partners who would otherwise be tender and respectful may become aggressive if they misinterpret their date's actions during heavy making out and heavy petting.

❖

"I think I've always been careful not to force myself on anyone," Jacoby, eighteen, comments. "But I've been with girls who, I'd say, pushed things to the point where I got so turned on I was going crazy. Then all of a sudden, they're like, 'Stop!' When that happens, it's all you can do to keep cool and back off. It makes me mad when girls push you and tease like that."

❖

Heavy petting is a poor idea for teenagers because passion and the sexual urge are so entwined. Before you and your date make out, it's important to talk ahead of time about how far you want the making out to go. Although talking about sex is awkward, you'll both end up feeling more comfortable with each other if you honestly talk about what you want and don't want.

❖

There's no easy way to talk about making out or sex, but you might try something like this:

"This is hard for me to talk about, but I feel like you and I know each other well enough to discuss something kind of serious. I think you're a great person. Otherwise I wouldn't be here. But we're getting to the point—physically—where we need to talk. It might be easy for us to get carried away—you know what I mean.

But I don't want that to happen. I won't feel right about it. I've decided to wait until I'm a lot older. I need to know if that's going to be okay with you—if you're comfortable with the way I feel. I'd really like to know what you think."

chapter 14
....

How to Say No

A teenager named Brad explains, "My girlfriend and I went through this whole thing last weekend because we were getting pretty carried away and I wanted to slow down and she thought that meant I didn't dig her. Thought she was ugly or something. When all I said was, 'Let's cool it and go out for a walk.' " [1]

One girl said when she tells a boy to stop, "He'll act like I was talking about the weather or something. He just keeps on going, as if I didn't mean what I said." [2]

A boy comments, "It's like a game. My friends told me that when a girl says no, she doesn't really mean it. So if a girl tells me quietly to stop and doesn't yell loud about it or hit me over the head with it, I'm not supposed to listen. It's a game to find out if she really means it." [3]

A young woman says, "I look at girls who haven't had sex and I'm jealous. It's like they control themselves, they can say no." [4]

IMAGINE THIS CHAIN OF EVENTS: A GUY OR GIRL YOU'VE HAD YOUR EYE on finally shows an interest in you. You go out a couple of times. You're excited and flattered. Your date is complimentary and affectionate and makes you feel special. It's a wonderful feeling, and you think you may be in love. But all of a sudden, they're clearly pushing you to have intercourse. You don't feel ready for sex, but you're afraid you'll lose them if you don't go along with it. You're confused. How do you say no?

Saying no is hard for lots of reasons. First of all, you don't know that much about the psychology of the opposite sex. (Reading chapter 3 will help.) Second, you're not that skilled in communicating how you feel, and talking about it seems terribly uncomfortable. Also, you may want desperately to be liked or loved, and you don't want to blow your chance.

A girl named Lena says, "You're scared the guy will think you're this incredible prude and he'll never want to go out with you again. You don't really want to have sex, but you're afraid he won't like you if you say no. You can't figure out what to do, so you just go along with it."

It can be hard for a boy to say no to a girl's pressure for sex because he doesn't want to appear unmanly or uncool.

It's especially hard for girls to say no because society teaches girls, more than boys, the importance of keeping the peace, of being agreeable and getting along well with others, and of not hurting anyone's feelings. In addition, females are often brought up to believe they should let males dominate them. Unfortunate-ly, this way of thinking makes it hard for a girl to say no to a boy.

Too often both sexes say yes, but later, they wish they'd said no.

A test of character and courage

Saying no to your partner can be a test of character and courage. It can be stressful and awkward, but it sure beats the guilt and pain you'll suffer if you realize later that you've done something you weren't ready for—something you may feel bad about for a long time.

❖

While you certainly don't need to apologize or make excuses for your decision to say no, you may want to let your partner down easy. In fact, in one survey of teenage girls, 84 percent said that what they most wanted to learn from sex education was how to say no without hurting their partner's feelings. [5]

❖

If you really like your boyfriend or girlfriend and are concerned about their feelings, you might say, "I do care for you, but I'd rather just be with you and talk with you than have sex."

❖

So a boy won't see it as a personal rejection, a girl could say, "I like you more than anybody I've dated, but I just don't want to have sex at this time in my life. If you care about me, I know you'll respect my decision." This lets him know she likes him a lot, and it makes her decision clear. She doesn't have to give any more reasons—it's her body and her life.

❖

If a girl pressures a boy, he could let her down easy with: "I know that sex can mess up a girl's life in lots of ways, and I respect you too much to let you get hurt that way."

Speak plainly

Letters to columnist Abigail Van Buren offer this advice:

> *Dear Abby:*
> *I'm a teen-aged girl getting ready to enter college, and I've had plenty of experience saying no. The most important thing to remember when you say no is to really mean it. Be completely serious, and if you have to, leave the location. You'd be surprised how many guys understand when you say no.*
> *This is probably what your parents and teachers have already told you. It's all true; it really works. But only if you speak plainly.*
> *—Saying No in Hampton, Va.*

> *Dear Abby:*
> *My ex-boyfriend asked me for sex on many occasions, and every time I had the same answer: "No." How did I do it? By sticking up for myself and what I believe in; by knowing I didn't have to if I didn't want to; by realizing I was not prepared for such an intimate relationship; and by asking myself, "Do I really want this?"*
> *Some advice for other teens like me: If you're doing it for him, because he supposedly wants to show his love for you, don't even think about it. Don't sacrifice yourself for his satisfaction. It's not worth it.*

Now some advice for parents: Please, talk to your daughters about sex. Tell them they don't need to do it with a guy to prove their love. We need your assurance more than anything. You may use my name.

—Daisy Yokley [6]

Dear Abby:

I'm twenty-four years old. I've been pregnant and have also had an STD. I know firsthand how difficult it is to say "no." It's not a matter of being rude. It's a fear of not being liked if you don't have sex, not being aggressive enough to refuse, and wanting someone to make you feel "loved." Abby, it's scary to say no, especially if you have low self-esteem. But I've finally learned to do it.

Sometimes I still feel self-conscious—and scared, too. But that's natural. What's not natural is being sixteen or seventeen or eighteen and being alone and pregnant or having AIDS.

It's OK to be rude if you have to be, and it's also OK to say "no." If you feel like you can't say "no," that's when you have to muster up your self-confidence and say, "Who cares if this person doesn't like me? I like myself enough to refuse!"

—Say Yes to Yourself in Minnesota [7]

❖

According to sex educator Carol Cassell, "If the other person cares about you as the unique person you are, they won't pressure you. If they can't honor your feelings and your decision to wait, you have learned a lot about them—they weren't someone worth being close with." [8]

Practice your responses

Push yourself hard to overcome shyness and embarrassment so that you can stand up for your decision.

Find a clear and kind way of saying no that you're comfortable with. Then practice it out loud. Think of what your date might say to try to talk you into changing your mind. Practice different responses. For example, if your date says, "You would if you loved

me," a girl could say, "If you loved *me*, you wouldn't pressure me."
A boy could respond to a girl's pressure by saying, "Sex can cause a
lot of problems. I value what we have together too much to risk it."

❖

Never have sex just because you can't figure out how to get out of
it. If you can't think of anything else, just say, "No. I'm not ready,"
or "No. It's not a good idea." Stick to it, repeating it over and over
in exactly the same words if your date continues to pressure you.
By using the same words over and over like a broken record, you
show the other person that their arguments are having no effect on
you. This makes them give up.

❖

Just because you say no to your partner's pressure to have sex
doesn't mean your relationship has to come to an end. As long as
you value each other, the two of you should be able to get past
this admittedly uncomfortable event. In fact, by showing your
respect for each other you can strengthen the relationship. If saying no means the end, then your respect was not mutual.

❖

A girl shouldn't be shocked if her boyfriend tries to push her further than she's comfortable going. He probably doesn't have any
more experience with these things than she does. He may think it's
his duty as a guy to push her. Many boys are grateful when their
girlfriends set limits—even though they may not act like it.

Don't feel "obligated" to have sex

When young women at a California abortion clinic were questioned, many said they had felt "obligated" to have sex.[9] Girls
need to remember they are under no obligation to have sex, no
matter how much they have made out with a boy and no matter
how much he may have spent on the date. So that she won't feel
she "owes" him sex, a girl can tell the boy that she'll pay for the
date next time; then she should do it.

❖

Many girls these days insist on paying their share of date expenses just because they don't want to feel they "owe" anything. But
even if a girl hasn't paid, she doesn't owe sex for money. That's
what prostitutes do.

❖

A guy's "reward" for a date is a girl's company—not sex.

❖

Just because your date is excited by you doesn't mean you're responsible for providing them with sex.

❖

At some high schools, prom night is sex night. Some young people of both sexes expect to have sex. But some girls feel pressured into it because their dates may have spent a small fortune on tickets, tux rental, photos, flowers, etc. If they haven't contributed financially, girls may feel pushed to contribute sexually.

❖

On prom night, some young people who really haven't made up their minds yet about sex find themselves caught up in the moment and end up doing something they later wish they hadn't.

Teens need to think over their values and be sure of themselves before prom night. If you believe in holding off on sex until you're older, your best date is someone who shares your values.

Don't get into a debate

If a boy tries to get a girl into an argument about her refusal to have sex, it's a bad idea for her to argue or debate. By getting into a back-and-forth argument, she may be giving him the impression that she could be persuaded. She should tell him, "I don't think you'd like it if I argued and pressured you into doing something you didn't think was right, so I would appreciate you not pressuring me." After that, a simple, firm "No, I'm not ready for that" should be enough. Then she should repeat it strongly— like a broken record—if he argues.

❖

If a boy grabs her, she should pull away without a hint of hesitation and yell "No!" She shouldn't get involved in playful struggling—the boy may think this is a turn-on. [10]

❖

If he's a more aggressive boy, a girl needs to be prepared to hear comebacks like "Why are you so uptight?" "What's wrong with you?" or "A real woman wouldn't stop now." These lines are designed to confuse a girl. If a guy uses these lines, it shows he has no respect for a girl's feelings. Why should a girl even date a boy who doesn't respect her and would hurt her if he could?

❖

Surveys have shown that boys are less likely to pressure a girl they love and respect. They are more likely to be concerned about her feelings and well-being and to want to protect her—not push her into sex. Girls should remember, a boy who REALLY loves you won't push.

Is your partner just using you?

If your girlfriend or boyfriend keeps pressing you to do something you're not ready for, it may be painful for you to accept, but there's a good chance they're trying to use you. They may be saying, "I love you," but what they're really doing is trying to exploit you for sex.

❖

A partner who argues that having sex will prove your love is really saying "I love it," not "I love you."

❖

A sixteen-year-old comments, "There's a lot of men out here who will try to sweet-talk you. You just have to ignore that stuff, because they will say they love you right up until it's time for you to have sex with them. As soon as you open up your legs for them, they don't want anything to do with you anymore. You have to be aware of those things." [11]

❖

Candy, seventeen, explains what happened after she carefully thought over her boyfriend's requests to have sex and decided against it. "So all of a sudden, this guy stopped calling me—this guy who had been all along telling me how much he loved me and everything. I didn't really feel bad about his not calling me anymore, because I knew that if sex was all he wanted, then I really didn't want to go out with him." [12]

❖

"Girls kick guys around, too," says Wiley, seventeen. "You might kid yourself that some girl likes you, but then you figure out that she's hoping for another notch on her gun. Some girls want to sleep with a bunch of guys, and they drop you if you don't perform."

❖

If you find yourself in the position of having to choose between losing a boyfriend or girlfriend and being pushed into sex, it's time to rush to the nearest exit. There is a better partner out there—one who's interested in the real you. You don't stand the slightest chance of finding them if you're in bed with Miss or Mr. Wrong.

❖

If you believe that your partner will leave you unless you agree to have sex, your relationship is already doomed. Having sex would be a very short-term "fix" and will only lead to a broken heart, or something worse.

❖

Sex is never a test of love.

❖

Compare these two relationships:

Relationship #1

First Partner: "I'll love you more if we make love. These feelings I have for you are so strong. You're so incredible. Making love is a beautiful way I can express the way I feel about you."

Second Partner [thinking silently]: "I might be rushing into this, but maybe my partner really will like me more if we do it. Maybe it will deepen our relationship. God, I hope this is a good idea. . . ."

Second Partner [aloud]: "Okay, if you're really sure you're serious about us."

Relationship #2 (quoted from a newspaper article in which the writer interviewed a real-life young couple who are determined to save sex for marriage)

First Partner: "There is so much more to her than just a sexual dynamic. I admire her intellectually. I know that sounds geeky and cheesy, but I'm serious. I love the way she has a tender heart. The way she gives to people. The way she cares about me and others. There is an openness and honesty that attracts me, that keeps me interested, that makes me want to know more. She's incredible."

Second Partner [in response to his comment]: "That's really, really rare. It's so nice to know that someone is interested in me and not my body. I see that as very strong and masculine of him. I admire that strength. It's a reminder to me of how strong his character is." [13]

Which kind of relationship would you want? Which relationship has the best chance of lasting? Why?

Lines That Partners Use

Here are some of the lines that some people use to try to talk their partners into sex:

- "You would if you loved me."
- "Everybody's doing it."
- "What's wrong with you? Are you frigid or something?"
- "If you don't help me, I'll get blue balls."
- "I'll make sure you don't get pregnant."
- "I'll love you more if we do it."
- "If you don't, it's all over between us."
- "Please, just this one time!"
- "Being a virgin is so old-fashioned."
- "You're so uptight. Why don't you just relax? You'll love it."
- "I just can't stop now."
- "Don't worry. I'll marry you if you get pregnant."
- "What's the matter? Don't you trust me?"
- "You're missing out on something incredible!"
- "What are you afraid of? Don't be a baby. A real woman/man would do it."

How girls can respond

More often, it's boys who try to talk girls into sex. Here are some lines that guys use and ways girls can respond. (Keep in mind, though, that a simple, forcefully stated "No. I don't want to" should be enough):

You would if you loved me.

If you loved me and respected my feelings, you wouldn't pressure me to do something I'm not ready for.

You must not really love me.

My decision is based on how I feel about sex, not how I feel about you. I prefer showing my love in other ways.

I'll leave you if you don't.

It looks like you care more about sex than you do about me. I'd like to go home now.

Everybody's doing it.

Then surely you can find somebody else to do it with, because I'm not ready.

If you really love me, prove it.

Sex doesn't prove you're in love. Respecting each other's feelings does. Please respect mine.

Aw, come on. I'll wear a condom.

My decision is not to have sex, and no matter what you say, I won't change my mind. Now, let's talk about something else!

How boys can respond

If a girl pressures a guy, he can use any of the following responses:

Everybody's doing it.

Don't you think we should get to know each other better? I do.

It will make our relationship even stronger.

Sex won't make our relationship stronger. In fact, it may ruin everything.

Don't worry—we can use a condom.

No method of birth control is sure. If you got pregnant, neither of our lives would ever be the same. And what about the baby's life?

You would if you loved me.

You're too smart to be acting like this—at least I always thought you were.

What are you afraid of? A real man would do it.

I don't think people should push each other into something that's such a big deal. So back off. What's your hurry?

You're missing out on something incredible!

We've got our whole lives ahead of us. I'd hate to mess up now.

It's a free country. It's a dangerous world.

Flirting can be fun, but sometimes it can be dangerous. If a girl is flirting, sending certain signals with her eyes, her voice, her clothing, or her body, a guy may think she's telling him she wants to have sex. She could even be risking assault. Sure, we live in a "free country" and you can act sexy and dress as scantily as you want, but we also live in a dangerous world. When a girl dresses or behaves in a certain way, guys may get a message she didn't intend.

About clothes, sex educator Teri Lester writes, "In a sense, clothes are the way we package ourselves. It's how we show who we are, what we think of ourselves. Usually, people put the most important aspect of a product on the package. If we see a package with chocolate on it, what do we expect to find inside? Chocolate, right? We are attracted to it if we like chocolate. If you dress in clothes that emphasize your sexuality, what does that say to others about your priorities? Who's going to be attracted to you? Are you interested in the kind of person who's focused on sex? Do you want to build a relationship with someone who's primarily interested in your body? What do your clothes say about you? Do they show that you have self-respect? Do they show that you take pride in your personal dignity? You can wear . . . vibrant, exciting clothes, without ever wearing the sort of thing that draws cheap attention." [14]

Fashionable behavior

Actress Jennifer Tilly says she's found that it helps to dress the way you want to behave. She found that when she dressed in low-cut tops and wacky outfits, she behaved "like a party girl." But Tilly says she's learned that when she dresses with more class and sophistication, she tends to behave like a classy sophisticate. [15]

Dating an older guy sounds cool, until . . .

If a girl dates an older boy, she should be prepared for someone who's more preoccupied with sex and more insistent on getting it than boys her age. Some older boys may even expect to have sex after dating a girl several times. Dating an older guy sounds cool until you're in his car or apartment and he's insisting on sex and you're feeling uncomfortable and threatened.

What's this about "blue balls"?

"Blue balls" describes pain in the testicles that some boys supposedly feel from having a prolonged erection. One of the oldest lines guys use is "You've got me so turned on, I've got 'blue balls.' We've gotta make love! This pain is unbearable!"

Is there even such a thing as having "blue balls"? Although it is possible for a boy to feel a slight ache in his testicles, it is certainly nothing serious and will go away harmlessly. But some girls fall for this line. Because they've kissed a boy and may have engaged in some petting, they feel guilty that perhaps the guy really got so turned on that he'll be in real pain if he can't finish The Act. This is baloney. Not having sex when you're turned on never hurt anyone.

❖

If a girl has sex just to make her partner feel better, she's cheating herself. She doesn't owe her virginity to anyone.

"No" means no, no matter what

Guys need to remember that a woman's "no" must be respected at any point in petting or making out. If a guy doesn't respect it, he can be charged with rape or attempted rape.

Introduce him to your folks (and other suggestions)

A girl should introduce her date to her parents before going out. If a guy meets her folks, he may act more responsibly and respectfully.

❖

Talk with your girlfriend or boyfriend ahead of time about how far you want to go. If you both understand and agree, you can relax. (See the end of chapter 13.)

❖

What if you're double-dating, you park, and the other couple starts seriously making out? If you don't want to feel pressured to do the same, try to remove yourself from the situation by suggesting that your date and you take a walk (only if the area is safe) or grab a bite at a nearby restaurant. Your date may be as grateful as you are to be removed from an awkward situation.

❖

Don't let your date talk you into going to a house where there are no adults present.

❖

Think about what might tempt you to say yes to sex. Decide if these reasons are good. Think about what could happen to you if you said yes, and think about how you might feel about it later. Decide what your Personal Policy about sex should be (see chapter 11).

What about teenage sex, drinking, and drug use?

Can drugs or drinking turn your teen dream date into a teen wolf? Some teenagers drink heavily or use drugs. The well-behaved date that you begin the evening with may be a very different person after a few hours of drinking or drug use. Among the problems you could face are dangerous driving, aggressive sexual advances, and an unwillingness to hear the word "no." Steer clear of the teen who drinks or uses drugs.

❖

Using drugs or having "one too many" drinks muddies your judgment and weakens your will to say no. Instead of making wise choices, teens end up having sex—often without using birth control or disease protection. Alcohol and drug use are connected with up to 80 percent of unplanned teen pregnancies and thousands of new cases of STDs. If you're drinking, you're not thinking.

❖

Some teens use drinking or drugs as a source of courage to talk themselves into sex before they're ready. Some foggily remember their "first time" as a real waste.

❖

Austin, eighteen, says he's still upset about something that occurred the year before between him and a girl who was just a friend. The two got drunk and started making out. "Neither of us meant for anything to happen, but we started kissing, and we didn't stop, and things just got way too intense. We ended up sleeping together. I think if we hadn't been drunk, we wouldn't have done it. She hasn't looked at me the same since, and I feel really bad about it. And then there's that whole thing about your 'first time.' I always wanted my first time to be something special, but it wasn't. I barely remember it."

❖

A young woman named Jane explains, "Everybody is so mixed up [about sex] that they just get drunk and do it. They try not to think about it the next day." [16]

Not playing with a full deck

Susan, a senior, says, "It's happened to me. Guys will try to get you to drink or to have a toke or whatever, and . . . you feel more relaxed and what they're saying to you doesn't seem as crazy. You don't say to yourself, 'Oh, I would never do that,' like you would if you were sober or playing with a full deck. And they start talking to you and you think, 'This guy digs me—he really wants to be with me.' And you're just not as careful as you should be." [17]

Wasted on prom night

It's become common for kids to drink themselves stupid or semi-conscious on prom night. These partygoers are taking an awful risk with their bodies and their futures. Some get so wasted that they don't even remember much about this special event—except how incredibly hung over and sick they were the next day. For a few, the most memorable souvenir of prom night is an unwanted pregnancy, an STD, or a heavy dose of shame.

Alcohol and abuse

While alcohol and drugs make it hard for most teens to think clearly and stick to their values, it makes some others become downright abusive. A boy could face violence or verbal intimidation from an out-of-control partner. A girl could face date rape.

chapter 15

....

Date Rape

Rape victim: "I cry myself to sleep and wake up in a cold sweat after reliving it all." [1]

Another recalls, "I tried to forget that it even happened for a long time. It was just one of the worst experiences of my life. It was awful, it was really frightening. The guy was much, much older than myself, and I felt that he really had power and control over me. It was without my consent." [2]

ABOUT ONE-THIRD OF RAPE VICTIMS ARE BETWEEN ELEVEN AND SEVENTEEN years old. [3] Rape is sexual intercourse against the will of the victim. In one study, 92 percent of teenage rape victims said they were acquainted with their attackers. [4] This kind of rape is called acquaintance rape, or date rape.

Some boys think that when a girl says "no" she means "maybe." They think a male's job is to push the girl until she gives in or changes her mind. They mistakenly think that because she enjoyed making out or petting, she's open to sexual intercourse. Even if she protests loudly, they may find her struggles sexually stimulating. If they overpower her and force her to have intercourse, it's rape. Date rape is a crime.

Every day in the U.S., more than 5,000 women are assaulted by men they know. [5] In a society where boys are pushed to separate sex from love, respect, and affection, the stage is set for date rape. Some boys see sex as a conquest, something to be taken from a girl. Girls, on the other hand, are socialized to be polite and "lady like" and to do as men ask. This kind of thinking leads to date rape. It is estimated that nearly half of all girls may experience rape or attempted rape. [6]

"It happens to more of us than anyone could guess," says one teen victim of date rape.

Boys may not know it's rape

Many boys do not understand that forcing their date to have sex against her wishes is rape. A survey of 114 college men found these results:

- "I like to dominate a woman." (91.3 percent)
- "I enjoy the conquest part of sex." (86.1 percent)
- "Some women look like they're just asking to be raped." (83.5 percent)
- "I get excited when a woman struggles over sex." (63.5 percent)
- "It would be exciting to use force to subdue a woman." (61.7 percent)[7]

❖

In another survey, one out of twelve college men admitted that they had forced or tried to force a woman to have sex with them. This constitutes rape and attempted rape, yet none of these men labeled themselves as rapists.[8]

❖

Even if a boy believes that a girl's confusing behavior led to the rape, he can be criminally prosecuted. Even if a girl's attacker is a friend or acquaintance, she should report this crime to the police.

Some guys plan their attacks

Some boys plan their attacks ahead of time. They may pick shy, unpopular girls who feel flattered to have been asked out. These boys don't think of themselves as rapists; they think they're out for fun. These rapists are often repeat offenders who've gotten away with it in the past.

❖

Date rape is rarely a simple crime of passion. It is often a boy's way of making himself feel powerful and strong.

❖

A boy NEVER has the right to force a girl to have sex:
- No matter how much money he's spent on her
- No matter if he feels she led him on
- No matter how long they've dated
- No matter if the two engaged in petting
- No matter if she is drunk or stoned
- No matter how seductively she is dressed

Think ahead

Sometimes a girl is uncertain in her own mind about how far she wants things to go. She may act seductively at first and let a boy go further and further while she makes up her mind. When she finally says no, he is angry. If he is an especially aggressive boy, he may tell himself that he has been misled and "deserves" satisfaction. If he forces her to have sex against her will, she can prosecute—but it's little consolation if she's been raped. Girls need to be careful not to send their dates confusing sexual signals.[9]

❖

If a boy is pushing his date beyond her sexual comfort zone and doesn't seem to hear her say "no," she needs to be very firm. She might say, "I don't enjoy this. Stop right now!" or "Take your hands off me, or I'm leaving." If he persists, he may be shocked into stopping if she says, "Leave me alone. This is rape!" She should not worry about making a scene. She may need to protest loudly. And she should not worry about being polite. If she's polite, a guy may think she just needs more persuading.[10]

❖

If he won't give up, she can try yelling, punching, and kicking. Then she should try to escape if she can.

❖

If a young woman feels that her date might beat her up or harm her even more if she doesn't agree to sex, she can try distracting him, playing for time, always looking for an opportunity to escape.

Lines to get you up to his place

Many rapes occur in the boy's house or apartment. A girl should keep in mind that going there alone with him can be dangerous. She should be suspicious of lines he may use to get her to come back to his apartment or house. He may say:

- "What are you so worried about?"
- "I promise I don't bite."
- "There's a great view from my place."
- "We'll only go upstairs for a drink."
- "I just forgot my jacket."
- "How can I ask you out again if you don't trust me?"

Her response to any of these lines could be "No, I don't want to. It's not a good idea." She should repeat this like a broken record if her date keeps insisting. Any decent guy will respect her reluctance to be put in a questionable situation.

Avoid these situations

Here are a few suggestions to help girls avoid situations that could put them at greater risk of date rape:

- Refuse to go to a secluded place. Tell your date that under any circumstances such an isolated place can be dangerous for both of you.
- If you end up at an empty house unexpectedly, strongly insist on leaving immediately. Don't worry about hurting the boy's feelings. Any time a girl expresses herself firmly to a boy, he can see that she respects herself and is no pushover.
- Be very clear with your date about what you want and don't want to do.
- Don't go to parties at the homes of people you don't know.
- Don't go to parties if parents won't be home.
- Carry extra change for emergency phone calls, and make sure you have a foolproof way to get home on your own.

- Be honest with your parents about who you'll be with and where you're going. If things get out of control and you need their help, you don't want to be afraid to call just because you'll be caught in a lie.
- If a party is getting out of hand, leave. Drug use, heavy drinking, and sexual assault go hand in hand.
- Don't get drunk or stoned.

❖

GIRLS SHOULD BE EXTREMELY CAUTIOUS ABOUT DATING GUYS WHO ARE SEVERAL YEARS OLDER—they are much more likely to insist on sex.

❖

A girl can end up sorry if she assumes that a rebellious, mysterious, wild, or "different" guy is going to be a cool date. His values may be quite different from hers, and she could end up in serious trouble. She should stick with guys who share her values.

Drinking, drugs, and date rape

Alcohol and drugs are often linked to date rape. If a girl has too much to drink and passes out, and if a boy then has sex with her, it's rape.

❖

If a guy is drunk and forces his date to have sex, being drunk is not a legal defense against the charge and prosecution of rape.

❖

If a girl gets drunk, her judgment may be so confused that she may not even realize she is in a potentially dangerous situation.

❖

Girls should remember: Lots of boys assume that a girl who's willing to get drunk or stoned is a good bet for sex.

What about the victim's feelings?

If a girl has been raped by a date, she may experience guilt or shame and feel stupid. She may not tell her parents because she fears they will be angry or will punish her. This is unfortunate, because she needs to be consoled, and she needs serious help. She should tell an adult—her parents, a doctor, minister, rabbi, counselor, a friend's parent—someone she can trust to be helpful and understanding.

Date rape victims should contact rape crisis centers

Counselors will help them deal with their emotions, teach them ways to avoid rape, and help restore their confidence.

❖

Even if a girl is reluctant to report the rape, it is very important that she have a medical examination as quickly as possible. She should be checked for possible injury and monitored for pregnancy and STDs. Evidence from this exam could help prosecute the attacker. A physician advises, "Don't clean up or change clothes before getting examined. This can destroy important evidence."

❖

A rape victim should not blame herself. She may have been foolish, naive, or not careful enough, but the rape is her attacker's fault, not hers.

A letter to the rapist

If a girl is raped by her date, the Association of American Colleges Project on the Status and Education of Women suggests that, in addition to seeking immediate medical attention and contacting a rape crisis center, the victim should write her attacker a letter. The letter should include dates, facts, feelings, and expectations.[11] This helps the victim feel she has taken constructive action, and it lets the attacker know how badly his actions have harmed the victim.

Dear John,

On June 21, after you took me to the movies, you invited me to your room to see the photos of your vacation. I thought you were someone I could trust. I didn't mind when you kissed me, but when you started pulling off my clothes, I told you to stop, but you didn't. You wouldn't listen to me and you wouldn't let me go. I was so afraid when you raped me. It was horrible, and I'm still so upset I can't sleep. I can't go to class, and I can't get it out of my mind. I cry all the time. I hate you and think you're disgusting. I never want to see you again, and I worry that you might do this to some other girl.

A special note for boys

If you commit date rape and your victim reports the attack, you could end up in jail. If you commit date rape and she doesn't report the attack, that's not the end of it. You will feel your own guilt and shame for the rest of your life knowing that you have forever harmed your victim's emotional and physical well-being.

❖

If you rape a girl, you damage her heart and soul. You damage her mother, her father, her brothers and sisters, her friends, and her future husband. She will remember this terrifying, degrading event with horror until the day she dies. She may have flashbacks and recurring dreams of the rape and will suffer depression and intense feelings of vulnerability. It can take many years to recover. One out of three rape victims considers killing herself. Eight out of ten say they will never be the same.

For more information

If you want more information on date rape and resisting attack, there is much useful information in public libraries as well as on the Internet. Every date rape is different, and there is a broad range of unforeseeable circumstances and possible responses. It is quite possible that, in certain situations, date rape cannot be avoided. The suggestions in this chapter are intended to be informative, but they are in no way offered as a guarantee or foolproof strategy for avoiding and dealing with date rape.

chapter 16

Sexually Transmitted Diseases:

One false move and you're infected

"I always thought of myself as a clean person. I shower every day. My girlfriend was clean. In fact, she was beautiful. But she gave me gonorrhea. I couldn't believe it. Now I feel dirty, like I'm infested with bugs or something."

"I hadn't known Tim very long, but he was such a gorgeous guy, I let myself go. I thought about using some kind of protection, but what was I supposed to do—stop everything and order him to put on a condom? He probably would have gotten mad. I was on the Pill anyway. So it just seemed easier to forget it. A month later, I found out I had genital warts. It's been horrible."

A young girl explains, "I could swear I never had any sign that I had a disease down there. No irritation, no pus— nothing! Then I started having this awful pain in my stomach. I tried to ignore it but it got so terrible I had to see a doctor. I was really sick. She said I had chlamydia, that I'd probably had it a long time without knowing it. It infected me deep inside, and now I may never be able to have kids. I still can't believe this happened to me."

MORE THAN TWENTY-FIVE DISEASES ARE SEXUALLY TRANSMITTED. Sexually transmitted diseases (STDs) spread from one person to another during sexual intercourse or close body contact—contact

157

involving the penis, vagina, rectum, or mouth. The Sexual Revolution has brought about an epidemic of STDs.

STDs spread faster among teenagers than any other group. Any teen—rich, poor, black, white, city or country dweller—can get an STD. STDs can make you very sick, can kill you, and can make you unable to have children. They can be transmitted to babies during childbirth, causing blindness, retardation, and death. Many teens with STDs have no idea they are infected and, therefore, do not seek treatment. They continue, unknowingly, to spread these diseases.

Some STDs can be treated and cured. Some cannot be cured. Some are developing a resistance to antibiotics. Some STDs cause sores in your genital area that give HIV / AIDS an easy entry point into your body.

Every year, three million teenagers get an STD. If you are sexually active, there's a fifty-fifty chance you'll get an STD by age twenty-five.[1]

It is estimated that one out of four sexually active teenage girls has an STD.[2] Women catch these diseases more easily than men due to body differences. During unprotected intercourse with an infected partner, women are twice as likely to catch some STDs, including chlamydia and gonorrhea.[3]

Because STDs are harder to detect in women, many women are unaware they are infected until their reproductive systems are so damaged that they can never have children.[4]

The younger the girl, the more susceptible she is to these infections. This may be because the cervix (the opening to the uterus) is immature and because the girl has fewer protective antibodies.[5]

There's no way to know if your partner is free from infection. They may not be truthful with you, may be too embarrassed to tell you, or may have a disease and not know it. In fact, your partner could have two sexually transmitted diseases at the same time and not know it.

The only sure way of protecting yourself against STDs is to abstain from vaginal, anal, and oral sex. If condoms with spermicides were used during every sexual intercourse by teenagers, they would provide fairly good protection, but it is a fact that many teens do not use condoms consistently. The most common reasons for not using condoms are discussed on pages 54 and 55. The following are a few of the most common STDs.

Chlamydia

Chlamydia is the number one STD in the U.S. Each year there are four million new cases—that's 11,000 new cases every day! The chlamydia microorganism can attack the reproductive systems of both men and women. Many victims have no symptoms and don't seek treatment. They continue to infect others.

❖

Every year one out of seven girls and one out of ten boys is infected with chlamydia.[6]

❖

Chlamydia symptoms may include burning, itching, discharge from the vagina or penis, burning urination, abdominal or lower back pain, fever, and pain and swelling in the testicles. Seventy-five percent of women and 25 percent of men have no symptoms until this infection has caused serious complications.[7]

❖

Chlamydia damages the reproductive systems of both young men and women and can cause sterility or infertility—the inability to have children in the future. Chlamydia can lead to infections of a girl's cervix and fallopian tubes (the tubes where sperm meets egg), causing scarring, infertility, and sterility.

❖

Chlamydia can lead to pelvic inflammatory disease (PID—discussed below), a serious and painful illness. Victims can end up with ongoing, long-term pelvic pain. PID can cause infertility and ectopic pregnancy.

❖

An ectopic pregnancy occurs when the fertilized egg implants someplace other than the uterus—usually a fallopian tube. The fertilized egg may begin developing in the tube. (This is called a tubal pregnancy.)[8] If left untreated, the tube will burst. This can result in the woman's death.

❖

Chlamydia infection can be transmitted from mother to infant during birth, leading to eye infection and possible blindness, pneumonia, and ear infections.

❖

While using condoms with spermicides will help prevent the spread of chlamydia, a very high number of sexually active teens do not use condoms, even though they know they should. Therefore, they are at great risk of catching and spreading this disease. You can eliminate your risk by abstaining from sex.

PID (pelvic inflammatory disease)

PID (pelvic inflammatory disease) affects a million women per year. The highest rate of infection is among teenagers. It is caused by different microorganisms, including gonorrhea and chlamydia, and can infect a woman's uterus, ovaries, and fallopian tubes.

❖

Symptoms include abdominal pain and tenderness, nausea, vomiting, chills, fever, and vaginal discharge and bleeding. Some women have no symptoms, but damage still occurs. Sexually active girls are at risk for this disease, which can be extremely serious, even fatal.

❖

PID causes inflammation and scarring of the fallopian tubes, which may lead to an ectopic pregnancy. This can be fatal. (See page 159.)

❖

A bad PID infection can require hospitalization and can cause sterility within a few weeks.

❖

Even though PID can be cured with antibiotics, it may already have caused irreversible damage to a girl's reproductive system before she begins taking antibiotics.

❖

Because sexually active teens often forget to use condoms or are too embarrassed to use them, they are at risk of getting PID. Teens who do not have sex are less likely to get a PID infection.

NGU (nongonococcal urethritis)

NGU (nongonococcal urethritis) is usually associated with male symptoms, but the organisms (such as chlamydia) that cause NGU can easily be transmitted to women.

❖

Boys with NGU may experience burning and itching around the opening of the penis, burning urination, and discharge from the penis. If untreated, NGU can lead to scarring of the urethra, causing problems with urination and ejaculation. Infection of the testicles can cause a boy to become sterile.

HPV (human papilloma virus)

Genital warts are caused by some types of HPV (human papilloma virus). Each year there are a million new cases of genital warts.

❖

Up to 90 percent of teens who have unprotected sex with an infected person will get HPV.[9] It may take as long as eight months for the warts to develop. They appear as hard, wrinkled, cauliflower-shaped bumps on the inner thighs, genital or anal areas. They can multiply quickly. They are treated with laser surgery, chemicals, and liquid nitrogen, but there is no real cure. The virus can lie dormant in the cells and cause recurrent flare-ups of warts.

❖

If an infant is exposed to HPV during birth, it is possible for the virus to lodge in the child's larynx, windpipe, and lungs, eventually causing serious breathing problems.

❖

Some types of HPV are linked to cervical cancer in women. Cervical cancer kills thousands of women every year. Some experts say that girls who become sexually active before eighteen are more likely to develop cervical cancer from HPV than women who postpone sex. One study of college women found that one out of four women developed some form of HPV within a year of becoming sexually active.[10]

❖

161

Generally, you can avoid HPV by avoiding skin-to-skin vaginal, anal, or oral sex. Condom use during intercourse is helpful, though not completely effective in preventing the transmission of HPV. The best way to keep from getting this disease is to abstain from sex.

Gonorrhea

Gonorrhea is highly contagious. There may be as many as three-quarters of a million teenagers with gonorrhea. Ninety percent of women with gonorrhea don't know they have it and unknowingly pass it on to partner after partner. Twenty percent of male victims are unaware they are infected.

❖

Symptoms may include discharge from the penis or vagina, burning urination, and, in girls, cramps and abnormal periods. But there may be NO symptoms.

❖

The gonorrhea bacterium can cause skin lesions, damage to the eyes, crippling arthritis, damage to the heart valves, and can result in stroke and heart failure. Gonorrhea can cause sterility in both sexes.

❖

In women, gonorrhea can result in pelvic inflammatory disease. (See "PID" on page 160.)

❖

Each year, 100,000 women in the U.S. are made sterile by gonorrhea.

❖

In men, gonorrhea can cause scarring in the urethra, which carries urine and semen to the penis. Painful ejaculation and extremely painful urination can result; later it may become impossible for the infected person to urinate. Even when no symptoms are present, the prostate and testicles can become badly infected, and sterility can result.

❖

Gonorrhea has been linked to cancer of the prostate in men. It can cause impotence (the inability to perform normal sexual intercourse).

❖

It is estimated that having gonorrhea increases the possibility of catching AIDS from an infected person by as much as 100 times. [11]

❖

The best way to avoid gonorrhea is to abstain from sexual activity. Condoms and spermicide will reduce the chance of spreading this disease, yet teens who know better often do not use protection.

Syphilis

Syphilis is called "a silent killer." It is caused by a highly contagious, spiral-shaped bacterium that enters the body, usually during sexual intercourse. It can also be transmitted by kissing, so NEVER kiss anyone with a sore on their mouth!

❖

The first sign of syphilis is a painless blister, or chancre, on the genitals at the site of entry. This chancre may develop a month after sexual intercourse and usually disappears within a few weeks. The victim may be unaware of its existence.

❖

During the second stage of syphilis, there may or may not be symptoms. Symptoms might include a sore throat, fever, headache, or skin rash. The victim might not think much of these symptoms.

❖

During the early part of the third stage of syphilis, there are no symptoms. In the following months and years, syphilis causes heart disease, blindness, deafness, paralysis, insanity, and death.

❖

Treatment for syphilis requires antibiotics. Some victims, unaware of their infections, go untreated.

❖

Babies can be infected with syphilis during childbirth, resulting in blindness, brain damage, and death.

❖

Condoms and spermicides used consistently are good protection against syphilis. However, the surest way for teenagers to avoid syphilis is to abstain from sex.

Herpes

Genital herpes is an incurable STD. One out of every five Americans over age twelve has herpes. The more sexual partners you have, the more likely you are to catch it. Sexually active teens are at great risk.

❖

Once herpes enters your body, it never leaves. You have it for life.

❖

Herpes is spread through vaginal, anal, or oral sex.

❖

It is often said that an infected individual can transmit the disease to a partner only when there is an active outbreak of herpes sores present. This is not true. The disease can also be transmitted in the twenty-four hours before the sores erupt, and the infected individual may be unaware that an outbreak is about to occur. Herpes can also be spread by carriers who have no idea they are infected.

❖

During an outbreak of herpes, the victim may experience inflamed skin, bumps or blisters in the genital area, pain, itching, burning, flu-like symptoms, swollen glands, muscle aches, headache, infection of the urethra, and burning urination. On average, herpes victims experience four recurrences of symptoms in a year. The virus may sometimes relocate to the buttocks. [12]

❖

During those periods when the victim has no symptoms, the herpes virus can reside at the base of the skull or spine. Outbreaks may be triggered by vigorous sexual activity, diet, stress, illness, and menstruation. [13]

❖

The use of condoms is not a guarantee of protection against herpes, because sores can be present in areas not covered by a condom.

❖

The presence of genital herpes sores makes it easier for HIV and other STDs to find an entry point in the genital area.

❖

In pregnant women, herpes causes an increased risk of premature birth and miscarriage. Infants born to mothers with herpes may suffer painful skin blisters, brain and organ infections, mental retardation, birth defects, and death. More than half of these babies are born to mothers who do not realize that they are infected with herpes. [14]

❖

Herpes affects its victims not only physically but also emotionally. Those infected may experience panic, fear, depression, and feelings of hopelessness and worthlessness.

❖

Considering the fact that forty million Americans have this disease, the only way for teens to eliminate their risk of catching it is to abstain from sex. Because of embarrassment, teenagers who are infected with herpes are not likely to tell their potential partners. They may use poor judgment about selecting times they think are safe for sexual activity. If they misjudge, they infect their partners.

Scabies and pubic lice

Scabies and lice are small insects that can be passed from one person to the next during close contact. They are highly contagious and can cause intense itching.

❖

Pubic lice look like microscopic crabs. They are bloodsuckers. Scabies burrow beneath human skin to lay eggs. Scratching these irritated areas can lead to other infections.

Shattered lives

There are thirteen million new STD cases in the U.S. every year. But this is only a statistic. It cannot describe the physical pain or feelings of despair and depression that STD victims experience.

❖

Later in life, when STD victims marry and try to begin a family, some discover that they are infertile, unable to have children. The diagnosis of infertility can threaten the survival of their marriage. One partner may feel angry and betrayed by the other. Both feel cheated out of their natural right to reproduce and care for a family.

❖

A woman writes to columnist Ann Landers describing the result of the "casual attitude" she once had about sex:

> *Dear Ann:*
>
> *I am a thirty-four-year-old married woman who is trying to become pregnant, but it doesn't look promising. All I have ever wanted in life was to be a mother, but I don't know if I will ever be able to have a child because of my past.*
>
> *When I was in college, I became sexually active. I slept with more men than I care to admit. . . . Somewhere in my wild days, I picked up an infection that left me infertile. . . . It seems the scar tissue damaged the inside of my fallopian tubes. . . . I am now married to a wonderful man who very much wants children, and the guilt I feel is overwhelming. . . . I am writing this letter with the hope that I can save others the heartache that I am going through.*
>
> *—Suffering in St. Louis* [15]

❖

Fifteen to 30 percent of U.S. couples who can't have children were made infertile by STDs. [16]

❖

Teens considering becoming sexually active should think very carefully about the risks of STDs—for themselves, for the baby that could result from an accidental pregnancy, and for their future marriage. By abstaining from sexual activity, you can avoid the heartache of sexually transmitted disease.

A few words about condoms

On pages 54 and 55, you read about some of the reasons why one-third of all sexually active teens don't use latex condoms consistently. Even though most teenagers know that pregnancy and disease are possibilities, they continue this risky behavior because they—like many teens—feel too guilty, embarrassed, shy, and uncertain to insist on condom use. They tell themselves that pregnancy and disease happen to other people, not them. A few thrill-seeking teens actually find sex more exciting because of the danger of pregnancy and disease and, therefore, choose not to use protection.

Any teen considering becoming sexually active should assume that they will be just as embarrassed and shy about condom use as so many other young people have been. They, too, are likely to skip protection at times, risking their future.

❖

But what about the teenagers who do purchase and use condoms? Can both partners feel safe? Not necessarily. Unless both partners are well educated about condom use, there can still be big problems. And the truth is, it is rare for both young teen partners to be knowledgeable about condoms.

❖

If you buy condoms, but have only a vague idea about how to use them, you may not be protected.

❖

Most teens and adults would be surprised to learn that condoms are only about 45 percent effective given the way teens use them, according to sex educator Ray Short. Teenage boys often purchase cheap condoms from vending machines, and they carry them in their wallets for months. The boy's movements—sitting down then standing up, over and over—eventually cause the tip of the condom, the most vital part, to rub and wear away. [17]

❖

Girls cannot assume or trust that their teen partner knows how to store a condom and use it properly.

❖

Columnist Ann Landers quoted Dr. Steven Sainsbury, a California physician, in a column dealing with condoms:

> My fifteen-year-old patient lay quietly on the gurney as I asked the standard questions: "Are you sexually active?" She said, "Yes." Next question: "Are you using any form of birth control?" The response was "No." Next question: "What about condoms?" Response, "No."
> Her answers didn't surprise me. She had a rip-roaring case of gonorrhea. It could easily have been AIDS. I treat teenagers like this one every day. Most are sexually active. Condoms are used rarely and sporadically.

Yet in the midst of the AIDS epidemic, I continue to hear condoms touted as the solution to HIV transmission. Condoms are being passed out in high schools, sold in college restroom dispensers and promoted on TV. The message is: Condoms equal safe sex.

As a physician, I wish it were true. It isn't. It is a dangerous lie.

Fact No. 1: In 1989, a survey among college women, a group we presume to be well informed on the risks of herpes, genital warts, cervical cancer and AIDS, showed that only 41 percent insisted on condom use. If educated women can't be persuaded to use condoms, how can we expect teenagers to do so?

Fact No. 2: Condoms fail frequently due to improper storage, handling and usage. The breakage rate during vaginal intercourse is 14 percent. For a person who averages sex three times a week, a 14 percent breakage rate equates to a failure nearly every two weeks.

For condoms to be the answer to AIDS, they must be used every time, and they can never break or leak. So what's the answer? The only answer is no sex until one is ready to commit to a monogamous relationship. The key words are abstinence and monogamy [sex only with one's marriage partner].

I can hear the moans. Condom fans murmur words like unrealistic, naive, and old-fashioned. Well, perhaps what is needed to stem the tide of AIDS and unwanted pregnancies is a return to those old-fashioned concepts.

To quote Dr. Robert C. Noble, a University of Kentucky infectious disease expert, "We should stop kidding ourselves. There is no safe sex. If the condom breaks, you may die." [18]

❖

Condoms are not foolproof. They are subject to misuse and breakage. They do not guarantee "safe sex," only "safer sex" when used properly. The only real guarantee teens have of eliminating their risk of unwanted pregnancy, AIDS, and other diseases is abstaining from sexual intercourse until they are older and in a life-long relationship.

PROBLEMS WITH CONDOMS

Here are a few of the problems teens encounter with condoms:

- Boys may not know exactly when to put on the condom and when to take it off. A condom should be applied as soon as the penis is erect. It should be removed immediately after ejaculation. The penis should be washed before further contact.

- Boys may not know how to put on a condom or how to keep it on, and many fumble and fail, sometimes right in the middle of intercourse.

- Boys, unsure of proper condom use, may go to their equally uncertain friends for information, instead of an adult or medical professional.

- Boys may not have practiced condom use ahead of time.

- Boys may have been drinking. Their judgment about condom use may be clouded, and they may be clumsy and less capable.

- Boys may handle the condom too roughly and tear it unknowingly.

- Boys may not know what conditions will damage a condom and make it susceptible to breakage. Some of these conditions include 1) body heat (when a condom is kept in a boy's wallet in his pants pocket); 2) use of non-water-based lubricants (such as Vaseline or hand lotion); 3) heat (when condoms are kept in the glove compartment of a hot car); 4) age (condoms deteriorate over time); 5) re-use (condoms should never be re-used); and 6) the use of lambskin, natural, or novelty condoms, which do not give full protection.

....

chapter 17

AIDS:

Sex in the Age of Death[1]

"I don't care if I die tomorrow as long as I have fun today." (Melinda, seventeen, chose this as her favorite quote for a personality sketch of herself on an Internet teen chat forum.)

"When I was nineteen, I took the HIV test on a whim," says twenty-year-old Ayisa. "I really didn't expect a positive result. But that's what it was. Everybody working at the clinic cried." [2]

Sister Kathleen, an AIDS volunteer, relates, "These are young people, gentle people. Beautiful young people who are dying much too soon. I've held them in my arms as they died. I've watched them as they fought to live. In my life, I've never seen such bravery." [3]

Tommy "The Duke" Morrison, a top heavyweight boxer, was diagnosed with HIV in 1996. When he announced his illness to the nation, he explained, "I was a big tough guy, thinking I was bulletproof. I considered myself pretty selective. I never really thought about [AIDS]. . . .[4] I knew the HIV virus was something that anyone could get, but I also believed that the chances were very, very slim. . . . I realize that there is a whole generation of kids out there like me that have totally disregarded the moral values that were taught to us by our parents, that somehow seem to treat sex as some kind of social activity rather than as a monogamous expression of love. . . .[5] I hope that I can serve as a warning that living this lifestyle can only lead to one thing, and that is misery." [6]

The following letter was written, but never sent, by beautiful, blond, trusting young Jennifer, who lived in a small Kansas town. She died in 1996, six years after contracting AIDS as a teenager.

Dear Dad,

This is the hardest letter I've ever written. I wish I could tell you in person. I have tried so many times. I just couldn't. Yes, dad, I have AIDS. . . .

The reason I couldn't tell you is because I didn't want you to hurt. That's the last thing I wanted to do. . . .

I don't want you to think I'm a bad person because I have this. I didn't get it from sleeping around or sharing needles. I've never ever done drugs.

I was so in love. I thought he would take care of me. I started dating him and I even told him to take an HIV test. He said it came up negative. I trusted and believed him. . . .

I was so shocked and hurt. How could it happen to me? . . .

You have seen how good I look. I'm not dying. I'm not sick. I'm healthy and I'm going to outlive you all. Please, please don't hate me. . . ." [7]

SEX CAN KILL. MOST TEENS DON'T WANT TO WORRY ABOUT AIDS. THE thinking may go, "It's too scary. Best to ignore it. It's a bummer that AIDS had to come along in my generation. I deserve my sexual freedom. It won't happen to me. Nobody I know has got it. We're safe at my school. So what if we don't use a condom? I'll be okay. Don't they have some kind of cure now for it anyway?"

It was this very kind of thinking that helped AIDS spread like wildfire through the homosexual population in the last two decades.

But AIDS isn't someone else's nightmare. If you're sexually active, it's YOUR nightmare.

What is AIDS and HIV?

AIDS (Acquired Immunodeficiency Syndrome) is the final and fatal stage of HIV infection. HIV stands for Human Immunodeficiency Virus. HIV can be transmitted through the exchange of bodily fluids during unprotected vaginal, anal, or oral sex. It may also be transmitted if an intravenous drug user shares a needle with someone infected with HIV.

❖

As soon as HIV enters the body, it begins making thousands, millions, then billions of copies of itself. This process goes on for many years. During this time—up to ten years or more—the victim looks fine, feels fine, and has no idea he or she is sick and will die. When this healthy-looking victim has unprotected sex with others during this period, those persons may contract HIV/AIDS.

❖

HIV destroys the immune system, making it impossible for the body to fight off other infections and cancers. These other diseases are what eventually kill the patient.

❖

When the person's immune system finally collapses, they may experience skin cancers, extreme weight loss, unexplained bleeding, coughing, terrible diarrhea, persistent herpes sores in the mouth and anus, exhaustion, mental problems, night sweats, fevers, rashes, pneumonia, and eventually death from infection.

❖

There is no vaccine or cure for HIV/AIDS. There are new treatments that give HIV sufferers hope, but with a price tag of up to $20,000 per year per victim, these treatments could cost the nation billions of dollars and will not be available to all. The price is just too high.

❖

The new drugs don't work for every patient. Up to one-third of patients show no improvement.

❖

It's possible that the new treatments will lose their effectiveness over time, as previous drugs have. A *Time* magazine article explained that the new strategy for HIV/AIDS treatment could backfire. According to the article, the virus could become less sensitive to medicines, and, consequently, patients might not respond to new drugs. Medicines might also cause a mutant AIDS strain to be created that would be even more resistant to treatment. A new "super HIV" might begin a devastating second AIDS epidemic.[8] This is, of course, a worst-case scenario that scientists hope will never happen.

❖

There are other reasons why the new treatments may not be the answer to AIDS. Dr. Jim Horton, a physician from North Carolina who treats HIV/AIDS patients, says there's no proof that these new drugs cure AIDS. The side effects of the medicine are so serious that some patients soon quit using them. Patients who stay on the drugs must carefully schedule their entire day around taking their pills. Patients on a normal HIV/AIDS treatment regimen may be taking up to thirty pills at carefully scheduled times throughout the day—with different requirements (on a full stomach, on an empty stomach, etc.). If patients begin missing doses, the drugs quickly lose their effectiveness.

Dr. Horton says it's dangerous thinking for teens to believe that these drugs lessen the seriousness of the AIDS epidemic.[9]

❖

Additional problems with the new treatment:

- The drugs should be started quickly after the person is infected. Yet most victims are unaware they're infected until much later.
- After a person has been infected for a few years (often without knowing it), the virus has found its way to the body's hiding places—the brain, lymph nodes, and testicles. The new medicines clear the virus from the bloodstream, but are not good at reaching these other hiding places.
- The new drugs can cause excruciating side effects, including kidney stones, nausea, cramping, diarrhea, spasms, and liver damage.

❖

Most states simply don't have the money to pay for these expensive treatments for so many victims. Some states have held lotteries for patients who could not afford the steep price of the drugs. The "winners" received treatment; the "losers" did not.

Teens are at great risk

Just being a teenager means you're in a high-risk group for AIDS. Other high-risk groups include IV drug users, prostitutes, and homosexuals. One of every four new AIDS infections occurs in a teenager. [10]

What would happen to your life?

If you got AIDS, what could happen to the quality of your life?

- HIV/AIDS patients quickly run out of money. Forget CDs, new clothes, or a car. AIDS victims are paying for medicine, doctors, and hospitals—fighting just to stay alive. They lose or can't get health insurance. AIDS patients may die penniless.
- They are sometimes deserted by friends and relatives who fear the disease.
- Almost no one wants to date or marry them because they're afraid of contracting AIDS themselves.
- Relatives may not want them to hug or kiss their children, even though such casual contact does not spread AIDS.
- They may never know the joys of the family life they might have had.
- Their careers may fall apart and they may lose their jobs.
- Other employers may be too afraid to hire them.
- If they have HIV dementia or mental problems, their bizarre behavior pushes others away.
- They may be terribly depressed.
- They may be lonely.
- They may suffer hair loss.
- They may lose their good looks.
- They may lose their sense of taste.

- They may feel dizzy.
- Some go blind.
- They are sickened by internal and external infections, everything from tuberculosis and pneumonia to rashes and skin ulcers.
- They have increasing thoughts and fears of death.

Why aren't teens more afraid of AIDS?

Why aren't teens more afraid of this terrible disease when they are in such a high-risk group? The biggest reason is that they just don't think it could happen to them. But, of course, it could. And it does.

❖

If you've never known anyone with HIV / AIDS, it's difficult to imagine you are at risk. The reason you don't see anyone your age sick with AIDS is that the virus lives and multiplies silently in the body for years. Kids you know right now may have HIV and show no symptoms and have no idea they are infected. Anyone they have sex with could be infected and, again, have no idea they were infected. Kids your age who contract HIV / AIDS will likely die when they are much older—even in their late twenties or thirties. That's why you may think you don't know any teens with HIV / AIDS.

❖

A young man named Jose explained, "My relationship with my parents is very, very close. My parents told me that I had to take care of myself, wear condoms, protect myself. . . . I'd say 'Yes, I'll be careful,' but I never paid any attention." [11]

Jose contracted HIV as a teenager and died in his early twenties in 1996 of AIDS complications.

❖

Young people assume their crowd of friends is "clean." But what if just one person in your group had sex with someone outside your group or school? One Indiana educator recalls how a young man came back from the army and infected seven junior high and high school girls.

❖

In Jamestown, New York, a young man infected twenty girls, some as young as thirteen, with the AIDS virus in 1997.

One of his victims explained that she was just looking for "someone to love me. . . . I was in love. I'd have done anything for him."

Another said, "He told me I was pretty, that I had a nice personality, stuff like that. . . . Having unprotected sex, I don't do it often unless I'm in love with someone."

❖

Another reason teens don't take AIDS seriously enough is that HIV-infected sports heroes like Magic Johnson and Tommy Morrison don't look sick. People are lulled into a false feeling that maybe HIV/AIDS isn't so terrible after all.

Whom can you trust?

Can sexually active teens trust that anybody is HIV-free? No. Your partner may not know that they're infected and may not be honest about past risky behaviors. Your partner might be too embarrassed to admit to multiple partners, same-sex partners, or needle use. In one study, half the young men and 40 percent of the young women said they would lie about the number of partners they'd slept with. Some males said they would lie to a girl and say they'd had a negative HIV test.[12]

❖

Is a negative HIV test really proof that your partner is not infected? No. An HIV test looks for antibodies in the blood, but it can take up to six months after initial infection for these antibodies to appear. If your partner takes an HIV test during the six months before the antibodies are present in the blood, the test could be negative—even though your partner does have HIV and can pass it on to you.

❖

Some unusual new HIV strains are not detected by current tests. Victims who do have HIV are told that their test result is negative.

What about condoms?

Consistent use of condoms is the best way that sexually active individuals can keep from getting HIV. But even the experts don't have complete faith in condoms. Some years ago at the National Conference on HIV, 800 physicians and other participants were asked to raise their hands if they would trust a condom to protect them during intercourse with a person known to have HIV. Not one hand was raised. The best protection is abstinence from sexual intercourse and other risky behaviors.

❖

Nearly half of the guys who say they have multiple sex partners say they rarely or never use condoms, according to a recent study in California. [13]

Only dirty people get AIDS. Right?

If your sex partner is clean and fresh, bathes daily, wears attractive clothing, and comes from a nice family, is it pretty safe to assume they don't have HIV? No. No matter how clean you are or how nice you look, you can catch HIV and transmit it unknowingly to others. Teens who think a condom is unnecessary during sex because their partner is clean and wholesome-looking are taking a big risk.

❖

Even though you and your partner begin a sexual relationship as virgins, if one of you has sex, even one time, with anyone else during your relationship, you could transmit HIV to the other partner. In a recent survey of college students from across the country, almost half confessed that they had cheated on their partner. [14]

Drinking and drugs make you more susceptible

Drinking and doing drugs not only impair your judgment so that you take risks you wouldn't ordinarily take, they also weaken your immune system. This makes you more susceptible to HIV infection.

It's easier for girls to catch AIDS

Girls are sixteen times more likely than guys to contract AIDS through heterosexual contact (intercourse with someone of the opposite sex). [15]

❖

In 1987, 14 percent of teen HIV cases were girls. But by 1994, girls made up 43 percent of teen cases. [16]

❖

Women with HIV can pass the virus to their babies during pregnancy, at birth, or while breastfeeding. Many babies with HIV/AIDS die by the time they're five years old.

❖

"I love my daughter so much. She's my whole world," says Adrienne, nineteen, who had a baby before she realized she was infected with AIDS. "But she's dying. Watching her get sicker and sicker is like having my heart ripped out."

❖

When you have completed your education and are ready to settle down, marry, and start a family, you will have lingering worries that you could harbor the HIV virus and could pass it to your innocent newborn if you have ever had unprotected sex. Who needs this kind of worry?

You can choose

Decisions about sex are truly life-and-death decisions. Not having sex is the most certain way for most teens to avoid HIV and sexually transmitted diseases.

❖

"There are only two kinds of people: those who are infected with HIV and those who might get it," says Dr. John G. Bartlett, a physician of infectious diseases. [17]

❖

Sex is no fun at all when you're dead.

chapter 18

If You're Smart . . .

Annie states, "I'm twenty-four years old and single. I have not ever entered into a sexual relationship with a man because I feel that's going to be my wedding gift to my husband. And the really neat thing is that when I explain that to guys that I date, they either drop me (because that's all they really wanted in the first place) or they begin to get really serious because virginity is becoming a very rare thing and that is a very special gift that you can only give once.

"I have eight female cousins, and every single one of them found 'the one' before they were eighteen, and had sex with them. Well, once is never enough, of course, and every single one of them were teenage mothers. Some of them married the father; some didn't. But as of now, they are all single parents, and have done very little with their lives. I, on the other hand, have been all over the world—New York, Hawaii, Boston, Florida, the Philippine Islands. . . .

"There are a lot of reasons to wait. Pick the one that you like best, but wait until you are ready to stay put and have lived a life before you do anything that could tie you down and make you wonder 'What if . . .' in twenty years." [1]

TODAY'S TEENAGERS ARE LED ON AND CONFUSED BY A CULTURE THAT displays sex everywhere for every possible commercial and entertainment purpose. Teens have been urged to wait, but they have not really been helped to understand WHY they should wait. They hear about "safe sex" but do not realize that rules for safe sex are no guarantee of a "safe" future.

If you have read this book carefully with an open mind, you have learned how teen sexual relationships can break hearts, erode self-confidence, and destroy romances. Sexually transmitted

181

diseases cause infection and death and prevent some teens from having children later on. In addition, teen sex brings hundreds of thousands of babies into the world whose futures are dismal. Teen parents find their own youth cut short and their prospects dimmed. Boys end up paying large sums of money to support children they may never see. Teenage sex prevents thousands of young people from living their dreams and achieving their goals.

If you wait until you're in your twenties—and hopefully in a lifetime relationship—before having sex, you will be better able to deal with the complex emotional issues of love and sexuality.

Those who say that youth is the happiest time of our lives must have forgotten how difficult the teenage years are. *The truth is that your happiest years lie ahead.* If you accept the challenges of getting a good education, making solid friendships, staying healthy, and learning how to combine love, respect, restraint, and responsibility, your future is bright.

What's the best thing that can happen to you in life? According to Basil and Elizabeth Williams, who have four children, eleven grandchildren, and eight great-grandchildren, "The best thing that can happen to a man and a woman is to share their lives together in marriage—helping one another through thick and thin, and depending on and trusting in one another. We have been each other's strength through war and peace, through sickness and health, for fifty-five years. We can only tell young people today to 'hang in there' for marriage and their lives will be rewarded more than they can imagine."[2]

Notes

Love and Sex

1. Carol Cassell, Ph.D., *Swept Away: Why Women Fear Their Own Sexuality* (New York: Simon and Schuster, 1987), 166, 130.

2. Associated Press, "Girls Are Motivated to Please Others, Survey Says," *Lawrence (Kansas) Journal-World* (April 9, 1996).

3. The Alan Guttmacher Institute, "Rethinking the First Time," *Family Planning Perspectives* (November–December 1997): 246. Based on an article from *The Journal of Adolescent Health* 21 (1997): 238–243.

4. Cynthia Akagi, *Dear Larissa: Sexuality Education for Girls 11–17* (Littleton, Colo.: Gylantic Publishing Company, 1994), 142.

5. Dan Habib, "Teen Sexuality in a Culture of Confusion," Knox Turner Associates (1995): http://www.intac.com/~jdeck/habib/ (January 2, 1997).

6. Abigail Van Buren, "Dear Abby," *Kansas City Star* (November 22, 1996).

7. Cassell, op. cit., 25.

8. Cassell, op. cit., 33.

9. Akagi, op. cit., 147.

10. Lewis B. Smedes, *Caring & Commitment: Learning to Live the Love We Promise* (San Francisco: Harper and Row Publishers, 1988).

How Sex Can Ruin Your Relationship

1. Lesley Jane Nonkin, *I Wish My Parents Understood* (New York: Penguin Books, 1985), 169.

2. Joyce Brothers, Ph.D., *What Every Woman Ought to Know about Love and Marriage* (New York: Ballantine Books, 1984), 52.

3. Matt Gibbon, "Teen Years 'The Best Time of Life?' Maybe, Once They've Passed," *Lawrence (Kansas) Journal-World* (February 22, 1996).

4. Bernard I. Murstein, *Love, Sex, and Marriage through the Ages* (New York: Springer Publishing Company, 1974), 386–387.

5. Anthony E. Wolf, Ph.D., *Get Out of My Life—But First Could You Drive Me and Cheryl to the Mall?* (New York: The Noonday Press, 1991), 171.

6. Steven Carter and Julia Sokol, *Men Like Women Who Like Themselves* (New York: Delacorte Press, 1996), 1–2.

7. Untitled, no author given, undated:
http://freeteens.org/love.power.txt/Missy.html, quoting Ann Landers column, web site accessed January 4, 1998.

Are Males and Females on the Same Sexual "Wavelength"?

1. "Relationship Games," *HomeArts Network Forum*, comment made November 25, 1996, The Hearst Corporation, copyright 1997:
http://homearts.com/cgi-bin/WebX?14@^273@ee6d45e/0 (March 14, 1997).

2. Anne Moir and David Jessel, *Brain Sex: The Real Difference between Men and Women* (New York: Carol Publishing Group, 1991), 103–104.

3. Ibid., passim.

4. David Popenoe, "Parental Androgyny," *Society* (September–October 1993): 8.

5. Barbara Dafoe Whitehead, "The Failure of Sex Education," *The Atlantic Monthly* (October 1994): 73.

6. Ronald F. Levant with Gina Kopecky, *Masculinity Reconstructed* (New York: Dutton, 1995), 234, discussing theories of B. Zilbergeld.

7. Ann Landers, "Teen-age Sex Is Risky Business," *Kansas City Star* (October 20, 1996).

8. Nonkin, op. cit., 158.

9. Nonkin, op. cit., 154.

10. Dr. Ruth Westheimer and Dr. Nathan Kravatz, *First Love: A Young People's Guide to Sexual Information* (New York: Warner Books, 1985), 32.

11. Whitehead, op. cit., 74.

12. Akagi, op. cit., 128–129.

13. Akagi, op. cit., 128.

14. Stefan Bechtel and Laurence Roy Stains, *Sex—A Man's Guide* (Emmaus, Pa.: Rodale Press, 1996), 438.

15. Archibald D. Hart, *The Sexual Man* (Dallas: Word Publishing, 1994), 70.

16. Nonkin, op. cit., 153.

17. John Bartlett, *Familiar Quotations*, 15th ed. (Boston: Little, Brown and Company, 1980), 347.

18. Robert Pasick, Ph.D., *Awakening from the Deep Sleep: A Powerful Guide for Courageous Men* (San Francisco: HarperSanFrancisco, 1992), 148–149.

19. John Munder Ross, Ph.D., *The Male Paradox* (New York: Simon and Schuster, 1992), 17.

"It Wasn't at All What I Expected"

1. Ruth Bell, *Changing Bodies, Changing Lives* (New York: Random House, 1980), 103.

2. Ibid., 103.

3. The Alan Guttmacher Institute, *Sex and America's Teenagers* (New York: The Alan Guttmacher Institute, 1994), 25.

4. Whitehead, op. cit., 73.

5. Bell, op. cit., 107.

6. Ann Landers, *Ann Landers Talks to Teen-Agers about Sex* (Englewood Cliffs, N.J.: Prentice-Hall, 1963), 35.

7. Howard R. and Martha E. Lewis, *The Parents' Guide to Teenage Sex and Pregnancy* (New York: St. Martin's Press, 1980), 102.

8. Nonkin, op. cit., 162–163.

9. Associated Press, "Girls Are Motivated to Please Others, Survey Says," op. cit.

10. Carol Cassell, Ph.D., *Straight from the Heart: How to Talk to Your Teenagers about Love and Sex* (New York: Simon and Schuster, 1987), 128–129.

11. Donald P. Orr, M.D., Mary Beiter, A.C.S.W., Gary Ingersoll, Ph.D., "Premature Sexual Activity as an Indicator of Psychosocial Risk," *Pediatrics* 87, no. 2 (February 1991): 141–147.

12. Joseph J. Piccione and Robert A. Scholle, "Combatting Illegitimacy and Counseling Teen Abstinence: A Key Component of Welfare Reform" (August 31, 1995):
http://www.savers.org/heritage/library/categories/healthwel/bg1051.html
(February 12, 1997).

13. Patricia Freeman, "Risky Business: One Day's Look at the Pleasures and Pressures of Sex at an Early Age," *People Weekly* (November 5, 1990): 53.

14. Judith Viorst, *Necessary Losses* (New York: Simon and Schuster, 1986), 131.

15. Nancy Friday, *My Mother, My Self* (New York: Delacorte Press, 1977), 270.

Pregnancy: It could happen to you

1. David Elkind, *All Dressed Up and No Place to Go: Teenagers in Crisis* (Reading, Mass.: Addison-Wesley Publishing Company, 1984), 131.

2. Carol Weston, *Girltalk: All the Stuff Your Sister Never Told You* (New York: Harper and Row Publishers, 1985), 94.

3. Allison Abner and Linda Villarosa, *Finding Our Way: The Teen Girls' Survival Guide* (New York: HarperCollins Publishers, 1995), 147.

4. Akagi, op. cit., 181.

5. Andrea Warren and Jay Wiedenkeller, *Everybody's Doing It* (New York: Penguin Books, 1993), 126.

6. James Leslie McCary, *Human Sexuality* (New York: Van Nostrand Reinhold Co., 1973), 81.

7. Gary Mucciolo, M.D., *Everything You Need to Know about Birth Control* (New York: The Rosen Publishing Group, 1990), 26.

8. The Alan Guttmacher Institute, op. cit., 30.

9. Lewis, op. cit., 178, quoting Judy Mage, Planned Parenthood counselor.

10. The Alan Guttmacher Institute, op. cit., 33.

11. Ellen Goodman, "Appendix is Pain in Dole's Side," *Lawrence (Kansas) Journal-World* (August 10, 1996), from study by Alan Guttmacher Institute.

12. Kathy Seymour Moore, "What's Love Got to Do with It?" *Family Planning Council of Western Massachusetts UPDATE* (Spring 1993): http://family.hampshire.edu/lorian.html (October 24, 1996).

13. Lewis, op. cit., 182.

14. Cassell, *Straight from the Heart*, op. cit., 181.

15. Weston, op. cit., 94.

16. The Alan Guttmacher Institute, op. cit., 52.

17. "Tragic: Teenage Pregnancies Too Often Result of Abuse by Adult Males," *The Wichita Eagle* (May 28, 1996).

18. Donna Ewy and Rodger Ewy, *Teen Pregnancy—The Challenge We Faced, the Choices We Made: Teens Talk to Teens about What It's Really Like to Have a Baby* (New York: Signet, 1984), 24.

19. Wilson W. Grant, M.D., *From Parent to Child about Sex* (Grand Rapids, Mich.: Zondervan Publishing House, 1973), 17.

20. Lewis, op. cit., 215.

21. "Teenage Pregnancy: Facts You Should Know" (The March of Dimes Birth Defects Foundation, 1994):
http://www.noah.cuny.edu/pregnancy/...ml#Health Risks to a Teenage Mother (July 28, 1996).

22. Bill Hewitt, et. al., "Mortal Choices at a Tender Age," *People Weekly* (July 23, 1990): 35.

23. Lynn Minton, "A Teenager Copes with Motherhood," *Parade Magazine* (April 7, 1996): 15.

24. Abner, op. cit., 162.

25. Robert C. Kolodny, Nancy J. Kolodny, Dr. Thomas Bratter, and Cheryl Deep, *How to Survive Your Adolescent's Adolescence* (Boston: Little, Brown and Co., 1984), 230.

26. Andy Silver, "I Got My Girlfriend Pregnant," *Sassy* (November, 1996): 33.

27. Kathy Seymour Moore, "Forgotten Fathers," *Family Planning Council of Western Massachusetts UPDATE* (Spring 1993):
http://family.hampshire.edu/jtpa.html (October 24, 1996).

28. Kolodny, op. cit., 229.

29. The Alan Guttmacher Institute, op. cit., 62.

30. Kolodny, op. cit., 229.

31. Elkind, op. cit., 7.

32. Ann Landers, "Teen Mother Shares Sorrow," *Lawrence (Kansas) Journal-World* (February 4, 1997).

33. "Built-in Risk for Teenage Pregnancies," *Science News* (May 27, 1995): 333.

34. "Teenage Pregnancy: Facts You Should Know," op. cit.

LISTEN UP, GUYS!
Eighteen years of child support is a long time!

1. Anne Browning Wilson, Attorney-at-Law, excerpt from address given at various high schools and junior highs in Kansas in the 1980s and 1990s.

2. Anne Browning Wilson, "If We Make A Baby, Do I Have to Pay?" a project of the Teen Pregnancy Coalition of Topeka/Shawnee County, Kansas, undated.

3. Associated Press, "Clinton: Welfare Moms Need to Name Child's Dad for Aid," *Lawrence (Kansas) Journal-World* (June 19, 1996).

4. Anne Browning Wilson, Attorney-at-Law, excerpt from address given at various high schools and junior highs in Kansas in the 1980s and 1990s.

Difficult Choices:
Options for the pregnant teen and her partner

1. Silver, op. cit., 33.

2. Ewy and Ewy, op. cit., 22.

3. Anna Quindlen, *Thinking Out Loud* (New York: Fawcett Columbine, 1993), 223.

4. Lewis, op. cit., 242.

5. Abner, op. cit., 157.

6. Silver, op. cit., 34.

7. Lewis, op. cit., 315.

8. Ann Landers, *Ann Landers Talks to Teen-Agers about Sex*, op. cit., 37.

9. The Alan Guttmacher Institute, op. cit., 60.

10. Elkind, op. cit., 133.

11. Ann Landers, "Ann Landers," *Boston Globe* (July 24, 1983).

12. Elkind, op. cit., 134.

13. David Boldt, "Yes, Daddies Do Matter," Knight-Ridder News Service, *Lawrence (Kansas) Journal-World* (April 3, 1996).

14. Ibid.

15. Elaine Kaplan, *Not Our Kind of Girl: Unraveling the Myths of Black Teenage Motherhood* (Berkeley: University of California, 1988), 93.

16. Carol Gilligan, *In a Different Voice: Psychological Theory and Women's Development* (Cambridge, Mass.: Harvard University Press, 1982), 123–124.

17. McCary, op. cit., 453.

18. Lewis, op. cit., 269.

19. Kolodny, op. cit., 229.

20. Associated Press, "Dolls Giving Teens a Lesson on Parenting," *Lawrence (Kansas) Journal-World* (December 16, 1996).

Is Everybody Doing It?
Peer pressure and self-esteem

1. Bell, op. cit., 100.

2. Ewy and Ewy, op. cit., 243.

3. William H. Masters, Virginia E. Johnson, and Robert C. Kolodny, *Masters and Johnson on Sex and Human Loving* (Boston: Little, Brown and Company, 1988), 145.

4. Bell, op. cit., 91.

5. Nonkin, op. cit., 80.

6. Habib, op. cit.

7. Mary Pipher, Ph.D., *Reviving Ophelia: Saving the Selves of Adolescent Girls* (New York: G.P. Putnam's Sons, 1994), 204.

8. "Abstinence: Pam Stenzel Brings 'Just Say No' Message to Schools," *Pro-Family News* (September 1996), quoting a suggestion by Pam Stenzel: http://www.mfc.org/pfn/9-96/Abstinence.html (January 5, 1997).

9. Alex Comfort and Jane Comfort, *The Facts of Love: Living, Loving, and Growing Up* (New York: Crown Publishers, 1979), 108.

10. Jeffrey Zaslow, "Never Be Afraid to Be Yourself," *USA Weekend* (October 11–13, 1996): 18.

11. Margaret Carlson, "A Girl's Best Friends," *Time* (January 22, 1996): 32, citing study showing that among 600 Best Friends members in Washington, D. C., 1.1 percent became pregnant over two years, as opposed to a citywide pregnancy rate of 24 percent for girls thirteen to eighteen.

12. Cheryl Wetzstein, "More Girls Say No to Sex with 'Best Friends' Help," *Washington Times* (January 16, 1996).

13. Abner, op. cit., 116.

14. Pipher, op. cit., passim.

15. Cassell, *Swept Away*, op. cit., 168.

What's the Double Standard?

1. Bell, op. cit., 67.

2. Nonkin, op. cit., 160.

3. Pipher, op. cit., 207.

4. Judy Mann, *The Difference: Growing Up Female in America* (New York: Warner Books, 1994), 183.

5. Bell, op. cit., 88.

6. Friday, op. cit., 271.

Sexual Liberation: Was it really liberating?

1. Julius Fast, *The Incompatibility of Men and Women and How to Overcome It* (New York: M. Evans and Company, 1971), 113.

2. Vance Packard, *The Sexual Wilderness: The Contemporary Upheaval in Male-Female Relationships* (New York: David McKay Co., 1986), 203.

3. Ibid., 201.

4. Kenneth Woodward and Betty Woodward, "Why Young People are Turning Away from Casual Sex," *McCall's* 101 (April 1974): 128.

5. Megan Marshall, *The Cost of Loving: Women and the New Fear of Intimacy* (New York: G.P. Putnam's Sons, 1984), 91.

6. Ibid., 92.

7. Whitehead, op. cit., 72–73.

8. "Ann Landers," *Lawrence (Kansas) Journal-World* (March 8, 1986).

Your Personal Policy on Sex

1. Cassell, *Straight from the Heart*, op. cit., 111.

2. Friday, op. cit., 274.

Why Choose Abstinence?

1. Derek Wojciech, "Giving the Gift (aka The Virginity 'FAQ')," Version 1.03A: http://osfl.gmu.edu/~dwojciec (March 9, 1996).

2. Nonkin, op. cit., 172.

3. David Plotz, "Just Don't Do It: A Young Couple Learns the Joys of No Sex," *Washington City Paper* (July 28, 1995).

4. Wojciech, op. cit.

5. Abner, op. cit., 139.

6. Laura Schlessinger, "Dr. Laura" column, *Kansas City Star* (January 19, 1997).

7. Lewis, op. cit., 49.

8. Kati Joyner, http://www.portoftacoma.com/CDHS/abstinence/sex (February 12, 1997).

9. Abigail Van Buren, "Dear Abby," *Kansas City Star* (November 7, 1996).

10. Bell, op. cit., 88.

11. Plotz, op. cit.

12. Habib, op. cit.

13. Ray E. Short, *Sex, Love, or Infatuation: How Can I Really Know* (Minneapolis: Augsburg Fortress, 1990), 102.

14. Ibid., 103.

15. Ibid., 110–111.

16. Ibid., 105.

17. Ibid., 103.

18. Ibid., 107–110, 116.

19. Ibid., 111–113.

20. Ibid., 111.

21. "How Long Should You Wait?," *HomeArts Network Forum,* comment made November 20, 1996, The Hearst Corporation, copyright 1997: http://home-arts.com/cgi/WebX?14@^38@ee6cbc9/0 (March 14, 1997).

22. Short, op. cit., 105–106.

23. Ann Landers, *Ann Landers Talks to Teen-Agers about Sex*, op. cit., 43.

24. Lynda Madaras, *The "What's Happening to My Body?" Book for Girls* (New York: Newmarket Press, 1988), 251–252.

There Are Many Other Ways to "Make Love"

1. Wojciech, op. cit.

2. Nonkin, op. cit., 154–155.

3. Nonkin, op. cit., 155.

4. Freeman, op. cit., 54.

5. Planned Parenthood, *How to Talk with Your Child about Sexuality* (Garden City, N.Y.: Doubleday and Company, 1986), 73.

6. Comfort, op. cit., 42.

7. Akagi, op. cit., 122.

How to Say No

1. Bell, op. cit., 92.

2. Bell, op. cit., 92.

3. Bell, op. cit., 92.

4. Nonkin, op. cit., 172.

5. John Leo, "Learning to Say No," *U.S. News and World Report* (June 20, 1994): 24.

6. Abigail Van Buren, "Self-respect Helps Girls Say No," *Kansas City Star* (September 18, 1996).

7. Abigail Van Buren, "Sometimes 'No' Just Can't Be Diplomatic," *Kansas City Star* (September 25, 1996).

8. Cassell, *Straight from the Heart*, op. cit., 214.

9. Lewis, op. cit., 79.

10. Lewis, op. cit., 92.

11. Abner, op. cit., 139.

12. Bell, op. cit., 100.

13. Plotz, op. cit.

14. Teri Lester, *Healthy Love: A Step-by-Step Method for Practicing Abstinence* (Overland Park, Kans.: RUC Publications, 1994), 18.

15. Knight-Ridder News Service, "Fashionable Behavior," *Kansas City Star* (October 26, 1996), quoting article in *USA Today Weekend*.

16. Pipher, op. cit., 205.

17. Bell, op. cit., 91.

Date Rape

1. Associated Press, "Rape Victims Find Comfort with E-mail Friendship," *Lawrence (Kansas) Journal-World* (April 21, 1996).

2. Habib, op. cit.

3. Pipher, op. cit., 219.

4. Jean O'Gorman Hughes and Bernice R. Sandler, " 'Friends' Raping Friends—Could It Happen to You?" Project on the Status and Education of Women, Association of American Colleges, (April 1987): http://www.cs.utk.edu/~bartley/ acquaint/acquaintRape.html (February 26, 1996).

5. Pipher, op. cit., 219.

6. Edwin M. Schur, *The Americanization of Sex* (Philadelphia: Temple University Press, 1988), 140.

7. Naomi Wolf, *The Beauty Myth* (New York: William Morrow and Co., 1991), 165.

8. Hughes, op. cit.

9. Ibid.

10. Ibid.

11. Ibid.

Sexually Transmitted Diseases:
One false move and you're infected

1. Lewis, op. cit., 152., quoting Dr. Walter Smartt, Los Angeles County Venereal Disease Control Division.

2. "Doing What Comes Naturally," *The Economist* 137 (November 17, 1990): 29.

3. The Alan Guttmacher Institute, op. cit., 30.

4. The Alan Guttmacher Institute, op. cit., 38.

5. The Alan Guttmacher Institute, op. cit., 31.

6. Jane Pratt and Kelli Pryor, *For Real: The Uncensored Truth about America's Teenagers* (New York: Hyperion, 1995), 191.

7. American Social Health Association, "Chlamydia," (Research Triangle Park, N.C.: American Social Health Association, 1990).

8. Eric Johnson, *Love and Sex in Plain Language* (New York: Harper and Row Publishers, 1985), 90.

9. Rita Baron-Faust, "Sexually Transmitted Diseases: Are You at Risk?" *McCall's* (April 1989): 108.

10. Paul Recer, "Panel: Cervical Cancer Preventable with Test," Associated Press, *Lawrence (Kansas) Journal-World* (April 4, 1996).

11. Gracie S. Hsu, "Suffer the Children: Title X's Family Planning Failure": http://www.townhall.com/townhall/FRC/insight/is95a5ab.html (August 24, 1996).

12. American Social Health Association, "Herpes" (Research Triangle Park, N.C.: American Social Health Association, 1994).

13. Ibid.

14. American Social Health Association, "Protect Yourself and Your Baby from Sexually Transmitted Disease (STD)" (Research Triangle Park, N.C.: American Social Health Association, 1991).

15. Ann Landers, "Wild Life Leaves Woman Scarred and Unable to Bear Children," *Kansas City Star* (October 3, 1997).

16. Hsu, op. cit.

17. Short, op. cit., 134–135.

18. Ann Landers, "Columnist Promotes Alternative to Unprotected Sex," *Lawrence (Kansas) Journal-World*, December 23, 1997, a reprint from her column of October 24, 1993, which contained an edited version of an article by Dr. Steven Sainsbury of San Luis Obispo, California, that appeared in the *Los Angeles Times*.

AIDS: Sex in the Age of Death

1. Simon Sebag Montefiore, "Love, Lies, and Fear in the Plague Years . . . (Sex in the 1990s)," *Psychology Today* (September–October 1992): 30.

2. Office of National AIDS Policy, "Youth & HIV/AIDS: An American Agenda—A Report to the President" (March 1996): 9.

3. Susan Kuklin, *Fighting Back: What Some People Are Doing about AIDS* (New York: G.P. Putnam's Sons, 1989: 47.

4. Eric Adler, "Athletes' Images Blur AIDS Horror," *Kansas City Star* (February 16, 1996).

5. David Boyce and Randy Covitz, "Wild and Crazy . . . and Careless," *Kansas City Star* (February 18, 1996).

6. David Boyce, "Morrison Takes Challenge," *Kansas City Star* (February 16, 1996).

7. Shirl Kasper, "No More Secrets," *Kansas City Star* (March 3, 1996).

8. Alice Park and Dick Thompson, "The Disease Detective," *Time* 148, no. 29 (December 30, 1996–January 6, 1997): 58.

9. Karen Garloch, "Beating the Odds," Knight-Ridder News Service, *Lawrence (Kansas) Journal-World* (December 10, 1996).

10. Office of National AIDS Policy, op. cit., passim.

11. Habib, op. cit.

12. Jerry Adler, et. al., "Safer Sex," *Newsweek* (December 9, 1991): 54–55.

13. Eric Adler, op. cit.

14. Tim Carpenter, "Survey Tabulates College Sex Horrors, Fantasies," *Lawrence (Kansas) Journal-World* (November 16, 1996), discussing study of 1,000 college students at twelve institutions, conducted for "American Journal" news program.

15. Dr. Carol J. Eagle and Carol Coleman, *All That She Can Be* (New York: Simon and Schuster, 1993), 171.

16. Office on National AIDS Policy, op. cit., 1.

17. "AIDS: What You Need to Know," (Middletown, Conn.: Weekly Reader Corporation, 1996), 3, quoting Dr. Bartlett, Chief, Division of Infectious Diseases, The Johns Hopkins Hospital, Baltimore, Maryland.

If You're Smart . . .

1. "Love and Marriage," *HomeArts Network Forum*, comment made February 7, 1997, The Hearst Corporation, copyright 1997: http://homearts.com/cgi-bin/WebX?14@^359@.ee72041/0 (March 14, 1997).

2. "Voices of the New Revolution," *In Focus Fact Sheet* (Washington, D.C.: Family Research Council).

Bibliography

Abner, Allison and Linda Villarosa. *Finding Our Way: The Teen Girls' Survival Guide*. New York: HarperCollins Publishers, 1995.

Acker, Loren E., Brian C. Goldwater, and William H. Dyson. *AIDS-Proofing Your Kids: A Step-by-Step Guide*. Hillsboro, Ore.: Beyond Words Publishers, 1992.

Adler, Eric. "Athletes' Images Blur AIDS Horror." *Kansas City Star* (February 16, 1996).

Adler, Jerry, et. al. "Safer Sex." *Newsweek* (December 9, 1991): 52–56.

"AIDS: What You Need to Know." Middleton, Conn.: Weekly Reader Corporation, 1996.

Akagi, Cynthia. *Dear Larissa—Sexuality Education for Girls 11–17*. Littleton, Colo.: Gylantic Publishing Co., 1994.

Alan Guttmacher Institute. *Sex and America's Teenagers*. New York, 1994.

Alter, Jonathan. "The Name of the Game is Shame." *Newsweek* 124 (December 12, 1994): 41.

Barbach, Lonnie, and David L. Geisinger. *Going the Distance*. New York: A Plume Book, 1991.

Baron-Faust, Rita. "Sexually Transmitted Diseases: Are You at Risk?" *McCall's* 116 (April 1989): 105–108.

Bartlett, John. *Familiar Quotations*. 15th ed. Boston: Little, Brown and Company, 1980.

Bechtel, Stefan, and Laurence Roy Stains. *Sex—A Man's Guide*. Emmaus, Pa.: Rodale Press, 1996.

Bell, Donald H. *Being a Man: The Paradox of Masculinity*. Brattleboro, Vt.: The Lewis Publishing Co., 1982.

Bell, Ruth. *Changing Bodies, Changing Lives*. New York: Random House, 1980.

Besharov, Douglas J. "Welfare: An Albatross for Young Mothers." *Wall Street Journal* (February 28, 1996).

Boldt, David. "Yes, Daddies Do Matter." Knight-Ridder News Service. *Lawrence (Kansas) Journal-World* (April 3, 1996).

Boyce, David. "Morrison Takes Challenge." *Kansas City Star* (February 16, 1996).

Boyce, David, and Randy Covitz. "Wild and Crazy . . . and Careless." *Kansas City Star* (February 18, 1996).

Brody, Jane E. "Guidelines for Parents of Teenagers Who Are, or Are About to Be, Sexually Active." *New York Times* (April 30, 1986).

Brothers, Dr. Joyce. *What Every Woman Ought to Know about Love and Marriage.* New York: Ballantine Books, 1984.

Brown, Lyn Mikel, and Carol Gilligan. *Meeting at the Crossroads: Women's Psychology and Girls' Development.* Cambridge, Mass.: Harvard University Press, 1992.

Buckley, William F., Jr. "Where's the Pressure?" *National Review* 40 (January 22, 1988): 73.

"Built-in Risk for Teenage Pregnancies." *Science News* 147 (May 27, 1995): 333.

Calderone, Dr. Mary S., and Dr. James W. Ramey. *Talking with Your Child about Sex.* New York: Random House, 1982.

Carlson, Margaret. "A Girl's Best Friends." *Time* (January 22, 1996).

Carpenter, Tim. "Survey Tabulates College Sex Horrors, Fantasies." *Lawrence (Kansas) Journal-World* (November 16, 1996).

Carter, Steven, and Julia Sokol. *Men Like Women Who Like Themselves.* New York: Delacorte Press, 1996.

Cassell, Dr. Carol. *Straight from the Heart: How to Talk to Your Teenagers about Love and Sex.* New York: Simon and Schuster, 1987.

———. *Swept Away: Why Women Fear Their Own Sexuality.* New York: Simon and Schuster, 1984.

Chambers, Carol A. *Child Support: How to Get What Your Child Needs and Deserves.* New York: Summit Books, 1991.

"Clinton: Welfare Moms Need to Name Child's Dad for Aid." Associated Press. *Lawrence (Kansas) Journal-World* (June 19, 1996).

Colson, Charles W. "Families Need a Dad; A Dad Needs Family." 1996 Religion News Service. *Kansas City Star* (June 15, 1996).

Comfort, Alex, and Jane Comfort. *The Facts of Love: Living, Loving and Growing Up.* New York: Crown Publishers, 1979.

"Condoms, Contraceptives, and Sexually Transmitted Disease." Research Triangle Park, N.C.: American Social Health Association, 1995.

Conine, Jon. *Father's Rights: The Sourcebook for Dealing with the Child Support System.* New York: Walker and Company, 1989.

Daly, Martin, and Margo Wilson. *Sex, Evolution and Behavior.* Boston: Willard Grant Press, 1983.

Daum, Meghan. "Safe-Sex Lies." *New York Times Magazine* (January 21, 1996): 32–33.

"Doing What Comes Naturally." *Economist* 137 (November 17, 1990): 29.

"Dolls Giving Teens Lesson on Parenting." Associated Press. *Lawrence (Kansas) Journal-World* (December 16, 1996).

Eagle, Carol J., and Carol Coleman. *All That She Can Be*. New York: Simon and Schuster, 1993.

Elkind, David. *All Grown Up and No Place to Go: Teenagers in Crisis*. Reading, Mass.: Addison-Wesley Publishing Company, 1984.

Ellis, Albert. *The American Sexual Tragedy*. New York: Lyle Stuart, 1962.

Ellis, Albert. *The Folklore of Sex*. Garden City, N.Y.: Country Life Press, 1951.

Ewy, Donna, and Rodger Ewy. *Teen Pregnancy—The Challenge We Faced, the Choices We Made: Teens Talk to Teens about What It's Really Like to Have a Baby*. New York: Signet, 1984.

"Fashionable Behavior." Knight-Ridder News Service. *Kansas City Star* (October 26, 1996).

Fast, Julius. *The Incompatibility of Men and Women and How to Overcome It*. New York: M. Evans and Co., 1971.

Fausto-Sterling, Anne. *Myths of Gender: Biological Theories about Women and Men*. New York: Basic Books, 1985.

Fleming, Anne Taylor. "Sex and Your Daughter." *Women's Day* 58 (February 21, 1995): 162.

France, Kim. "AIDS Explodes among Teens." *Utne Reader* (July–August, 1992): 30.

Freeman, Patricia. "Risky Business: One Day's Look at the Pleasures and Pressures of Sex at an Early Age," *People Weekly* 34 (November 5, 1990): 50–57.

Friday, Nancy. *My Mother, My Self*. New York: Delacorte Press, 1977.

Garloch, Karen. "Beating the Odds." Knight-Ridder News Service. *Lawrence (Kansas) Journal-World*. (December 10, 1996).

Gibbon, Matt. "Teen Years 'The Best Time of Life?' Maybe, Once They've Passed." *Lawrence (Kansas) Journal-World* (February 22, 1996).

Gibbs, Nancy. "Teens: The Rising Risk of AIDS." *Time* 138 (September 2, 1991): 60.

Gilligan, Carol. *In a Different Voice: Psychological Theory and Women's Development*. Cambridge, Mass.: Harvard University Press, 1982.

"Girls are Motivated to Please Others, Survey Shows." Associated Press. *Lawrence (Kansas) Journal-World* (April 9, 1996).

Goodman, Ellen. "Appendix is Pain in Dole's Side." *Lawrence (Kansas) Journal-World* (August 10, 1996).

Grant, Wilson W. *From Parent to Child about Sex*. Grand Rapids, Mich.: Zondervan Publishing House, 1973.

"Guides for Sexually Active Teens." New York Times News Service. *Lawrence (Kansas) Journal-World* (April 30, 1986).

Habib, Dan. "Teen Sexuality in a Culture of Confusion." Knox Turner Associates (1995). http://www.intac.com/~jdeck/habib (January 2, 1997).

Hamel, Marilyn. *Sex Etiquette*. New York: Delacorte Press, 1984.

Hamilton, Eleanor. "Other Kinds of Sex." http://www.ptreyeslight.com/prl/columns/hamilton (March 11, 1996).

Hart, Archibald D. *The Sexual Man*. Dallas: Word Publishing, 1984.

"Herpes." Research Triangle Park, N.C.: American Social Health Association, 1994.

Hewitt, Bill, Patricia Freeman, Margaret Nelson, and Bill Shaw. "Mortal Choices at a Tender Age." *People Weekly* (July 23, 1990): 30–35.

"HIV Infection and AIDS: Are You at Risk?" Centers for Disease Control and Prevention. U.S. Government Printing Office (September 1994).

"How Long Should You Wait?" *HomeArts Network*. The Hearst Corporation. Copyright 1997. http://homearts.com/WebX?14@^38@ee6cbc9/0 (March 14, 1997).

"HPV." Research Triangle Park, N.C.: American Social Health Association, 1995.

Hsu, Gracie S. "Suffer the Children: Title X's Family Planning Failure." http://www.townhall.com/townhall/FRC/insight/is95a5ab.html (August 24, 1996).

Hudson, Liam, and Bernadine Jacot. *The Way Men Think: Intellect, Intimacy and the Erotic Imagination*. New Haven, Conn.: Yale University Press, 1991.

Hughes, Jean O'Gorman, and Bernice Sandler. " 'Friends' Raping Friends— Could It Happen to You?" Project on the Status and Education of Women, Association of American Colleges (April 1987). http://www.cs.utk.edu/~bartley/acquaint/acquaintRape.html (February 26, 1996).

Janus, Sam. *The Death of Innocence: How Our Children are Endangered by the New Sexual Freedom*. New York: William Morrow and Company, 1981.

Johnson, Eric. *Love and Sex in Plain Language*. New York: Harper and Row, 1985.

Joyner, Kati. http://www.portoftacoma.com/CDHS/abstinence/sex (February 12, 1997).

Kantrowitz, Barbara. "Breaking the Poverty Cycle." *Newsweek* 115 (May 28, 1990): 78.

Kaplan, Elaine. *Not Our Kind of Girl: Unraveling the Myths of Black Teenage Motherhood*. Berkeley: University of California Press, 1997.

Kasper, Shirl. "No More Secrets." *Kansas City Star* (March 3, 1996).

Katchadourian, Herant. *The Biology of the Adolescent*. San Francisco: W.H. Freeman and Company, 1977.

Koff, Gail J. *Love and the Law*. New York: Simon and Schuster, 1989.

Kolodny, Robert C., Nancy J. Kolodny, Dr. Thomas Bratter, and Cheryl Deep. *How to Survive Your Adolescent's Adolescence.* Boston: Little, Brown and Company, 1984.

Kondracke, Morton. "Prude and Prejudice." *New Republic* 205 (August 5, 1991): 43.

Kreps, Bonnie. *Subversive Thoughts, Authentic Passions: Finding Love without Losing Yourself.* New York: Harper and Row, 1990.

Kuklin, Susan. *Fighting Back—What Some People Are Doing about AIDS.* New York: G.P. Putnam's Sons, 1989.

Landers, Ann. "Ann Landers." *The Boston Globe* (July 24, 1983).

———. "Ann Landers." *Kansas City Star* (October 20, 1996).

———. "Ann Landers." *Kansas City Star* (October 3, 1997).

———. "Ann Landers." *Lawrence (Kansas) Journal-World* (March 8, 1986).

———. "Ann Landers." *Lawrence (Kansas) Journal-World* (February 4, 1997).

———. "Ann Landers." *Lawrence (Kansas) Journal-World* (December 23, 1997).

———. *Ann Landers Talks to Teen-Agers about Sex.* Englewood Cliffs, N.J.: Prentice-Hall, 1963.

Leo, John. "Learning to Say No." *U.S. News and World Report* 116 (June 20, 1994): 24.

Leslie, Connie. "Amid the Ivy, Cases of AIDS: College Campuses Offer Students No Sanctuary." *Newsweek* 112 (November 14, 1988): 65.

Lester, Teri. *Healthy Love: A Step-by-Step Method for Practicing Abstinence.* Overland Park, Kans.: RUC Publications, 1994.

Levant, Dr. Ronald F., with Gina Kopecky. *Masculinity Reconstructed.* New York: Dutton, 1995.

Lewis, Howard R., and Martha E. Lewis. *The Parent's Guide to Teenage Sex and Pregnancy.* New York: St. Martin's Press, 1980.

"Love and Marriage." *HomeArts Network Forum.* The Hearst Corporation. Copyright 1997 (March 14, 1997).

Madaras, Lynda. *The "What's Happening to My Body?" Book for Girls.* New York: Newmarket Press, 1988.

Mann, Judy. *The Difference: Growing Up Female in America.* New York: Warner Books, 1994.

Marshall, Megan. *The Cost of Loving: Women and the New Fear of Intimacy.* New York: G.P. Putnam's Sons, 1984.

Masters, William H., Virginia E. Johnson, and Robert C. Kolodny. *Masters and Johnson on Sex and Human Loving.* Boston: Little, Brown and Company, 1988.

McCary, James Leslie. *A Complete Sex Education for Parents, Teenagers, and Young Adults.* New York: Van Nostrand Reinhold Company, 1973.

McCary, James Leslie. *Human Sexuality*. New York: Van Nostrand Reinhold Company, 1973.

McGough, Elizabeth. *Who Are You? A Teenager's Guide to Self-Understanding*. New York: William Morrow and Company, 1976.

Minton, Lynn. "A Teenager Copes with Motherhood." *Parade Magazine* (April 7, 1996): 15.

Moir, Anne, and David Jessel. *Brain Sex: The Real Difference Between Men and Women*. New York: Carol Publishing Group, 1991.

Montefiore, Simon Sebag. "Love, Lies, and Fear in the Plague Years. . . . (Sex in the 1990s)." *Psychology Today* 25 (September–October 1992): 30.

Moore, Kathy Seymour. "Forgotten Fathers." *Family Planning Council of Western Massachusetts UPDATE* (Spring 1993). http://family.hampshire.edu.jtpa.html (October 24, 1996).

———. "What's Love Got to Do with It?" *Family Planning Council of Western Massachusetts UPDATE* (Spring 1993). http://family.hampshire.edu/lorian.html (October 24, 1996).

Morical, Lee. *Where's My Happy Ending? Women and the Myth of Having It All*. Reading, Mass.: Addison-Wesley Publishing Company, 1984.

Mucciolo, Gary. *Everything You Need to Know about Birth Control*. New York: The Rosen Publishing Group, 1990.

Murstein, Bernard I. *Love, Sex, and Marriage through the Ages*. New York: Springer Publishing Company, 1974.

Nonkin, Lesley Jane. *I Wish My Parents Understood*. New York: Penguin Books, 1985.

Orenstein, Peggy. *School Girls: Young Women, Self-Esteem and the Confidence Gap*. New York: Doubleday, 1994.

Orr, Donald P., M.D., Mary Beiter, A.C.S.W., and Gary Ingersoll, Ph.D. "Premature Sexual Activity as an Indicator of Psychosocial Risk." *Pediatrics* 87, no. 2 (February, 1991): 141–147.

Packard, Vance. *The Sexual Wilderness: The Contemporary Upheaval in Male-Female Relationships*. New York: David McKay Co., 1968.

Park, Alice, and Dick Thompson. "The Disease Detective." *Time* 148, no. 29 (December 30, 1996–January 6, 1997): 56.

Pasick, Robert. *Awakening from the Deep Sleep: A Powerful Guide for Courageous Men*. San Francisco: HarperSanFrancisco, 1992.

Piccione, Joseph J., and Robert A. Scholle. "Combatting Illegitimacy and Counseling Teen Abstinence: A Key Component of Welfare Reform." (August 31, 1995). http://www.savers.org/heritage/library/categories/healthwel/bg1051.html (February 12, 1997).

Pipher, Mary. *Reviving Ophelia: Saving the Selves of Adolescent Girls.* New York: G.P. Putnam's Sons, 1994.

Pittman, Frank S., III. *Man Enough: Fathers, Sons, and the Search for Masculinity.* New York: G.P. Putnam's Sons, 1993.

Planned Parenthood. *How to Talk with Your Child about Sexuality.* Garden City, N.Y.: Doubleday and Company, 1986.

Plotz, David. "Just Don't Do It: A Young Couple Learns the Joys of No Sex." *Washington City Paper* (July 28, 1995).

Popenoe, David. "Parental Androgyny." *Society* 30 (September–October, 1993): 5–11.

Powell, Douglas. *Teenagers, When to Worry and What to Do.* Garden City, N.Y.: Doubleday and Company, 1986.

Pratt, Jane, and Kelli Pryor. *For Real: The Uncensored Truth about America's Teenagers.* New York: Hyperion, 1995.

"Protect Yourself and Your Baby from Sexually Transmitted Disease." Research Triangle Park, N.C.: American Social Health Association, 1991.

Quindlen, Anna. *Thinking Out Loud.* New York: Fawcett Columbine, 1993.

"Rape Victims Find Comfort with E-mail Friendship." Associated Press. *Lawrence (Kansas) Journal-World* (April 21, 1996).

Recer, Paul. "Panel: Cervical Cancer Preventable with Test." Associated Press. *Lawrence (Kansas) Journal-World* (April 4, 1996).

Reed, Susan. "Wake-up Call." *People Weekly* 42 (October 10, 1994): 103.

"Relationship Games." *HomeArts Network Forum.* The Hearst Corporation. Copyright 1997. http://homearts.com/cgi-bin/WebX?14@^273@ee6d45c/0 (March 14, 1997).

"Rethinking the First Time." *Family Planning Perspectives.* New York: Alan Guttmacher Institute. (November–December 1997): 246.

Rochlin, Gregory. *The Masculine Dilemma: A Psychology of Masculinity.* Boston: Little, Brown and Company, 1980.

Ross, John Munder. *The Male Paradox.* New York: Simon and Schuster, 1992.

Rubenstein, Carin, Ph.D., and Phillip Shaver, Ph.D. *In Search of Intimacy.* New York: Delacorte Press, 1974.

Schlessinger, Laura. "Dr. Laura." *Kansas City Star* (January 19, 1997).

Schur, Edwin M. *The Americanization of Sex.* Philadelphia: Temple University Press, 1988.

Scott, Sharon. *How to Say No and Keep Your Friends.* Amherst, Mass.: Human Resource Development Press, 1986.

Seligmann, Jean. "Condoms in the Classroom." *Newsweek* 118 (December 9, 1991): 61.

Sellner, James G., and Judith A. Sellner. *Loving For Life.* North Vancouver, British Columbia, 1986.

Sevetson, Martha. "Teen-birth Epidemic Tests Cowley County Resources." *Wichita Eagle* (July 12, 1993).

Sex Information and Education Council of the United States. *Sexuality and Man.* New York: Charles Scribner's Sons, 1970.

Shapiro, Laura. "Guns and Dolls." *Newsweek* (May 28, 1990): 56–65.

Short, Ray E. *Sex, Love, or Infatuation: How Can I Really Know?* Minneapolis: Augsburg Fortress, 1990.

Silver, Andy. "I Got My Girlfriend Pregnant." *Sassy* (November, 1996).

Smedes, Lewis B. *Caring & Commitment: Learning to Live the Love We Promise.* San Francisco: Harper and Row Publishers, 1988.

Smith, Manuel J. *Yes, I Can Say No.* New York: Arbor House, 1986.

"Social Costs of Teenage Sexuality." *Society* 30 (September–October, 1993): 3.

"Some Questions and Answers about Chlamydia." Research Triangle Park, N.C.: American Social Health Association, 1990.

"Some Questions and Answers about NGU." Research Triangle Park, N.C.: American Social Health Association, 1990.

"Some Questions and Answers about PID." Research Triangle Park, N.C.: American Social Health Association, 1990.

"STD (VD)." Research Triangle Park, N.C.: American Social Health Association, 1994.

Sternberg, Robert J. *The Triangle of Love: Intimacy, Passion, Commitment.* New York: Basic Books, 1988.

"Stopping Gonorrhea the Clap." Research Triangle Park, N.C.: American Social Health Association, 1994.

"Teenage Pregnancy: Facts You Should Know." The March of Dimes Birth Defects Foundation, 1994. http://www.noah.cuny.edu/pregnancy/...ml#Health Risks to A Teenage Mother (July 28, 1996).

"Tragic Teenage Pregnancies Too Often Result of Abuse by Adult Males." *Wichita Eagle* (May 28, 1996).

Van Buren, Abigail. "Dear Abby." *Kansas City Star* (September 18, 1996; September 25, 1996; November 7, 1996; and November 22, 1996).

Vaughan, Peggy, and James Vaughan, Ph.D. *"Sex Education: For Parents Only."* Copyright 1996. http://www.oeg.net/vaughan/sex.html (February 19, 1997). Quoting Jane Pauly in "Sex, Teens and Public Schools," PBS (October, 1995).

Viorst, Judith. *Necessary Losses.* New York: Simon and Schuster, 1986.

"Voices of the New Revolution." *In Focus Fact Sheet.* Family Research Council. Washington, D.C. Undated.

Warren, Andrea, and Jay Wiedenkeller. *Everybody's Doing It.* New York: Penguin Books, 1993.

Wattleton, Faye, and Elizabeth Keiffer. *How to Talk with Your Child about Sexuality.* Planned Parenthood. Garden City, N.Y.: Doubleday, 1986.

Weisman, Betsy, and Michael H. Weisman. *What We Told Our Kids about Sex.* San Diego: Harcourt Brace Jovanovich, 1987.

Westheimer, Dr. Ruth, and Dr. Nathan Kravatz. *First Love: A Young People's Guide to Sexual Information.* New York: Warner Books, 1985.

Weston, Carol. *Girltalk: All the Stuff Your Sister Never Told You.* New York: Harper and Row, 1985.

Wetzstein, Cheryl. "More Girls Say No to Sex with 'Best Friends' Help." *Washington Times* (January 16, 1996).

Whipple, Beverly, and Gina Ogden. *Safe Encounters.* New York: McGraw-Hill Book Company, 1989.

Whitehead, Barbara Dafoe. "The Failure of Sex Education." *The Atlantic Monthly* (October, 1994).

Wilson, Anne Browning. "If We Make a Baby, Do I Have to Pay?" Teen Pregnancy Coalition of Topeka/Shawnee County, Kansas. Funded by Kansas State Department of Education.

Wojciech, Derek. "Giving the Gift (aka The Virginity 'FAQ')" Version 1.03A (July 21, 1995). http://osfl.gmu.edu/~dwojciec (March 9, 1996).

Wolf, Anthony E., Ph.D. *Get Out of My Life—But First Could You Drive Me and Cheryl to the Mall?* New York: The Noonday Press, 1991.

Wolf, Naomi. *The Beauty Myth.* New York: William Morrow and Co., 1991.

Wolman, Benjamin B., ed., and John Money, consulting ed. *Handbook of Human Sexuality.* Englewood Cliffs, N.J.: Prentice-Hall, 1980.

Woods, Samuel G. *Everything You Need to Know about STD: Sexually Transmitted Disease.* New York: The Rosen Publishing Group, 1990.

Woodward, Kenneth, and Betty Woodward. "Why Young People Are Turning Away from Casual Sex." *McCall's* 101 (April 1974).

"Youth & HIV/AIDS: An American Agenda—A Report to the President." Office of National AIDS Policy (March 1996).

Zaslow, Jeffrey. "Never Be Afraid to Be Yourself." *USA Weekend* (October 11–13, 1996).

Permissions

page 7. Reprinted from *Swept Away: Why Women Fear Their Own Sexuality*, by Carol Cassell ©1987, Simon & Schuster, with permission from Carol Cassell.

page 10. Reprinted with permission from Dan Habib, from "Teen Sexuality in a Culture of Confusion," by Dan Habib © 1995, Knox Turner Associates: http://www.intac.com/~jdeck/habib/

page 12. Reprinted from *Swept Away: Why Women Fear Their Own Sexuality*, by Carol Cassell ©1987, Simon & Schuster, with permission from Carol Cassell.

page 21. Reprinted from *I Wish My Parents Understood*, by Lesley Jane Nonkin © 1985, Penguin Books, with permission from Lesley Jane Nonkin Seymour.

page 22. Reprinted from *What Every Woman Ought to Know about Love and Marriage*, by Dr. Joyce Brothers © 1984, Ballantine Books, with permission from Joyce B. Enterprises.

page 26. Reprinted from *Men Like Women Who Like Themselves*, by Steven Carter and Julia Sokol, © 1996, Delecorte Press, with permission from Dell Publishing Permissions Department.

page 28. Reprinted: permission granted by Ann Landers and Creators Syndicate.

page 31. Reprinted from "Relationship Games," http://homearts.com ©1997 The Hearst Corporation, with permission from the *HomeArts Network Forum*.

page 32. Reprinted from "Parental Androgyny" by David Popenoe, *Society Magazine*, September–October 1993. Reprinted with permission of Copyright Clearance Center.

page 33. Reprinted from *I Wish My Parents Understood*, by Lesley Jane Nonkin © 1985, Penguin Books, with permission from Lesley Jane Nonkin Seymour.

pages 34–35. Reprinted with permission from Gylantic Publishing—Akagi C. (1994). *Dear Larissa: Sexuality Education for Girls 11-17*. Littleton, CO. Gylantic Publishing.

page 37. Reprinted from *I Wish My Parents Understood*, by Lesley Jane Nonkin © 1985, Penguin Books, with permission from Lesley Jane Nonkin Seymour.

page 38. Reprinted with permission of Simon & Schuster from THE MALE PARADOX by John Munder Ross. Ross, John Munder, *The Male Paradox*, New York: Simon & Schuster, 1986.

page 39. From CHANGING BODIES, CHANGING LIVES by Ruth Bell. Copyright © 1980 by Ruth Bell. Reprinted by permission of Random House, Inc.

page 41. From CHANGING BODIES, CHANGING LIVES by Ruth Bell. Copyright © 1980 by Ruth Bell. Reprinted by permission of Random House, Inc.

page 41. Reprinted with permission from Ann Landers.

page 44. From "Risky Business," by Patricia Freeman, *People Weekly*, November 5, 1990. Reprinted with permission from PEOPLE.

page 44. Reprinted with permission of Simon & Schuster from NECESSARY LOSSES by Judith Viorst. Judith Viorst, *Necessary Losses*, New York: Simon & Schuster, 1986.

page 46. Reprinted from *My Mother, My Self*, by Nancy Friday, Delecorte Press, with permission from Dell Publishing Permissions Department.

page 49. Reprinted from *Finding Our Way: The Teen Girls' Survival Guide*, by Allison Abner and Linda Villarosa ©1995, with permission from HarperCollins Publishers.

page 49. Reprinted from *Everybody's Doing It*, by Andrea Warren and Jay Wiedenkeller © 1993, Penguin Books, with permission from the authors.

page 57. Reprinted from *Teen Pregnancy—The Challenge We Faced, The Choices We Made: Teens Talk to Teens About What It's Really Like to Have a Baby*," by Donna Ewy and Rodger Ewy © 1984, Signet, with permission from Donna Ewy.

page 57. From *From Parent to Child about Sex,* by Wilson W. Grant, © 1973, Zondervan Publishing House, with permission from Wilson W. Grant.

page 58. Reprinted from *The Parents' Guide to Teenage Sex and Pregnancy*, by Howard R. and Martha E. Lewis, © 1980, St. Martin's Press, with permission from St. Martins Press.

page 58. From "Mortal Choices at a Tender Age," by Bill Hewitt, et. al., *People Weekly,* July 23, 1990. Reprinted with permission from PEOPLE.

page 58. From "Fresh Voices"column by Lynn Minton (April 7, 1996), *Parade*. Reprinted with permission from *Parade*. Copyright © 1996.

pages 58–59. Reprinted from *Finding Our Way: The Teen Girls' Survival Guide*, by Allison Abner and Linda Villarosa ©1995, with permission from HarperCollins Publishers.

page 60. Reprinted: permission granted by Ann Landers and Creators Syndicate.

pages 64–67. Reprinted with permission from *"If We Make A Baby, Do I Have To Pay,"* by Anne Browning Wilson.

page 67. Reprinted with permission from the Associated Press.

page 69. Reprinted from *Teen Pregnancy—The Challenge We Faced, The Choices We Made: Teens Talk to Teens About What It's Really Like to Have a Baby,* by Donna Ewy and Rodger Ewy ©1984, Signet, with permission from Donna Ewy.

page 71. Reprinted from THINKING OUT LOUD, by Anna Quindlen, © 1993, Fawcett Columbine, with permission from Random House.

page 73. Reprinted from *Finding Our Way: The Teen Girls' Survival Guide,* by Allison Abner and Linda Villarosa © 1995, with permission from HarperCollins Publishers.

pages 76–77. Reprinted with permission from Ann Landers.

page 80. Reprinted from *Not Our Kind of Girl: Unraveling the Myths of Black Teenage Motherhood,* by Elaine Bell Kaplan ©1997, University of California Press, Berkeley, with permission from Elaine Bell Kaplan.

page 80. From IN A DIFFERENT VOICE by Carol Gilligan. Copyright ©1982 by Carol Gilligan. Reprinted by permission of Harvard University Press.

page 85. From CHANGING BODIES, CHANGING LIVES by Ruth Bell. Copyright © 1980 by Ruth Bell. Reprinted by permission of Random House, Inc.

page 85. Reprinted from *Teen Pregnancy—The Challenge We Faced, The Choices We Made: Teens Talk to Teens About What It's Really Like to Have a Baby,* by Donna Ewy and Rodger Ewy ©1984, with permission from Donna Ewy.

page 86. Reprinted from *Masters and Johnson on Sex and Human Loving,* by William H. Masters, Virginia E. Johnson, and Robert C. Kolodny Copyright © 1998, Little, Brown and Company, with permission from William H. Masters.

page 87. From CHANGING BODIES, CHANGING LIVES by Ruth Bell. Copyright © 1980 by Ruth Bell. Reprinted by permission of Random House, Inc.

pages 88–89. Reprinted with permission from Dan Habib, from "Teen Sexuality in a Culture of Confusion," by Dan Habib © 1995, Knox Turner Associates: http://www.intac.com/~jdeck/habib/

page 90. Reprinted by permission of The Putnam Publishing Group from REVIVING OPHELIA by Mary Pipher, M.D. Copyright © 1994 by Mary Pipher, M.D.

page 92. From "More Girls Say No to Sex with 'Best Friends' Help" (January 16, 1998). Reprinted from *The Washington Times*.

page 92. Reprinted from *Finding Our Way: The Teen Girls' Survival Guide*, by Allison Abner and Linda Villarosa © 1995, with permission from HarperCollins Publishers.

page 95. Reprinted from *Swept Away: Why Women Fear Their Own Sexuality*, by Carol Cassell ©1987, Simon & Schuster, with permission from Carol Cassell.

page 97. From CHANGING BODIES, CHANGING LIVES by Ruth Bell. Copyright © 1980 by Ruth Bell. Reprinted by permission of Random House, Inc.

page 97. Reprinted from *I Wish My Parents Understood*, by Lesley Jane Nonkin © 1985, Penguin Books, with permission from Lesley Jane Nonkin Seymour.

page 97. Reprinted by permission of The Putnam Publishing Group from REVIVING OPHELIA by Mary Pipher, M.D. Copyright © 1994 by Mary Pipher, M.D.

page 99. From CHANGING BODIES, CHANGING LIVES by Ruth Bell. Copyright © 1980 by Ruth Bell. Reprinted by permission of Random House, Inc.

pages 99–100. Reprinted from *My Mother, My Self*, by Nancy Friday, Delacorte Press, with permission from Dell Publishing Permissions Department.

page 101. Reprinted from "Why Young People Are Turning Away from Casual Sex," by Kenneth and Betty Woodward, *McCall's* 101 (April 1974), with permission from Kenneth Woodward.

page 101. Reprinted from *The Sexual Wilderness*, by Vance O. Packard © 1968, David McKay Co., Inc., with permission from Barbara L. Smith, Executrix of the Estate of Vance O. Packard.

page 101. From *The Incompatibility of Men and Women and How to Overcome It* by Julius Fast. Copyright © 1971 by Julius Fast. Reprinted by permission of the publisher M. Evans and Company, Inc., 216 East 49th Street, New York, NY 10017 USA.

page 102. Reprinted by permission of The Putnam Publishing Group from THE COST OF LOVING by Megan Marshall. Copyright © 1984 by Megan Marshall.

page 104. Reprinted: permission granted by Ann Landers and Creators Syndicate.

page 113. From "Giving the Gift (aka The Virginity 'FAQ'), version 1.03A: http://osfl.gmu.edu/~dwojciec, by Derek Wojciech, March 9, 1996, reprinted with permission from Derek Wojciech.

page 113. Reprinted from *I Wish My Parents Understood,* by Lesley Jane Nonkin © 1985, Penguin Books, with permission from Lesley Jane Nonkin Seymour.

page 113. From "Just Don't Do It: A Young Couple Learns the Joys of No Sex," by David Plotz, *Washington City Paper,* July 28, 1995, reprinted with permission.

pages 113–114. From "Giving the Gift (aka The Virginity 'FAQ'), version 1.03A: http://osfl.gmu.edu/~dwojciec, by Derek Wojciech, March 9, 1996, reprinted with permission from Derek Wojciech.

page 114. Reprinted from *Finding Our Way: The Teen Girls' Survival Guide,* by Allison Abner and Linda Villarosa © 1995, with permission from HarperCollins Publishers.

page 114. Passage from "Common Sense, Moral Values" reprinted with permission. Copyright © 1997, Dr. Laura Schlessinger. Distributed by *New York Times* Special Features/Syndication Sales.

page 116. From CHANGING BODIES, CHANGING LIVES by Ruth Bell. Copyright © 1980 by Ruth Bell. Reprinted by permission of Random House, Inc.

page 117. From "Just Don't Do It: A Young Couple Learns the Joys of No Sex," by David Plotz, *Washington City Paper,* July 28, 1995, reprinted with permission.

page 118. Reprinted with permission from Dan Habib, from "Teen Sexuality in a Culture of Confusion," by Dan Habib © 1995, Knox Turner Associates: http://www.intac.com/~jdeck/habib/

page 120. Reprinted from "How Long Should You Wait?," http://homearts.com ©1997, The Hearst Corporation, with permission from the *HomeArts Network Forum.*

page 122. From *The "What's Happening to My Body?" Book for Girls,* by Lynda Madaras with Area Madaras. Copyright © 1983, 1988 by Lynda Madaras. Reprinted by permission of Newmarket Press, 18 East 48th Street, New York, NY 10017.

page 123. From "Giving the Gift (aka The Virginity 'FAQ'), version 1.03A: http://osfl.gmu.edu/~dwojciec, by Derek Wojciech, March 9, 1996, reprinted with permission from Derek Wojciech.

pages 123–124. Reprinted from *I Wish My Parents Understood,* by Lesley Jane Nonkin © 1985, Penguin Books, with permission from Lesley Jane Nonkin Seymour.

page 128. From "Risky Business," by Patricia Freeman, *People Weekly,* November 5, 1990. Reprinted with permission from PEOPLE.

About the Author

Susan Browning Pogány has been a writer, editor, and photographer for over twenty-five years. Formerly with the Oregon Health Sciences University, Portland, she has won state, national, and international awards for medical and science writing, editing, and photography. She has also worked as a reporter for The Wichita Eagle/Beacon and as a photographer for the Massachusetts Institute of Technology.

Pogány studied at Northwestern University's Medill School of Journalism and graduated from NU in 1969 with a BA in English Literature.

The author is recognized as one of the country's finest artists specializing in marbled papers (decorative papers used in bookbinding). A special edition containing her original designs was presented by President Bill Clinton to President Boris Yeltsin of Russia at the Hyde Park–New York Summit in 1995.

Pogány is the wife of an organic chemist and the mother of two teenage sons. The family resides in Lawrence, Kansas.